AQUACISES

Restoring and Maintaining Mobility with Water Exercises

Miriam Study Giles

Mills & Sanderson, Publishers
Bedford, MA 01730

Published by Mills & Sanderson, Publishers
Box U, Bedford, MA 01730
Copyright ©1988 Miriam Study Giles

Library of Congress Cataloging-in-Publication Data

Giles, Miriam Study, 1920-

   Aquacises: restoring and maintaining mobility with water exercises.

   Bibliography: p.

   1. Aquatic exercises.   2. Exercise for the aged.
3. Physical fitness for the aged. I. Title.
RA781.17.G55 1988   613.7'1   87-35671
ISBN 0-938179-11-X

DEDICATION

To the Senior Water Exercise Group and Staff
Members of Mt. Rainier Swimming Pool,
22722 Nineteenth Avenue South,
Des Moines, Washington

CONTENTS

Conditioning and Stretching ... 101

Exercises (most with illustrations)

Other books by Miriam Study Giles

The Golden Link

A Novel Based on the Life of Mustafa Kemal,
1962

How to Write College Papers

A Manual of Style, 1967

AQUACISES

INTRODUCTION

Although I once had held swimming records and had been a featured ballet dancer, my get up and go had got up and gone. I hobbled painfully into the county swimming pool, and because of an old back injury that had become arthritic, I could hardly walk along the deck. After a couple of months my old swimming style returned and I was helping the young manager lead other young people's aquatic exercises. I wondered why fitness buffs were all young. Why couldn't people in their sixties (and over), like me, benefit from the magic that restores flexibility, endurance, and a sense of well-being? I started a class for "seniors," people from sixty to a tottering ninety. At first just three or four ladies parked their canes beside the pool, knelt at the top step, and were helped into the water. Now these same ladies jump into the water along with thirty to forty other seniors, men and women, who look like Rockettes while they move to music -- or simply to my hand clapping and enthusiastic directions and demonstrations.

I want to share these exercises and directions with the twenty-eight million four thousand other seniors in the United States (July 1, 1984, Statistical Abstracts of The U.S.) and give them a reliable handbook so that they can teach themselves what I teach to my classes. Study and practice of water exercises can promote psychological and physical fitness, social and safety benefits through body training -- exercises to develop and improve all physical capacities of the body while the participants are moving in, or are partially submerged in the water -- specifically related to the needs of senior citizens who do not need to know how to swim.

Aquacising is like a fountain of youth, only instead of drinking the water, you move in it. Except for those for whom partial immersion in water is detrimental, everyone can benefit from doing water exercises: the expert swimmer; the non-swimmer; most handicapped people; the very young, and senior citizens. Neither skill nor strength is necessary.

Most of these exercises are adapted and created from conventional calisthenics for being executed in the water. They strengthen the heart and improve circulation. They condition and tone all muscles, and they relax and help everyone. Aquacises are valuable for youthful and even competitive swimmers' conditioning, as their warming-up and tapering-off activities. They are especially valuable for those who do not swim and who want to become accustomed to the water. They help people overcome their fear of the water. They help teach basic aquatic skills that are a prerequisite for learning to swim. They also prepare, strengthen, and condition people for participation in other sports, in becoming trim and graceful in drama, dancing, and modeling.

On the other hand, everyone who begins any fitness program should first check with his physician to ascertain whether or not the activity is all right for him. For example, the approximately 25,000 people in the United States who have had laryngectomies or who breathe through a trachea tube or a stoma that goes directly to the windpipe in the throat, should be very cautious even in a bathtub or in the shower. Obviously, aquacises are not for them.

Except for those who are medically excluded, aquacising meets the needs of people who have various problems, such as disabilities of the spinal area, hemiplegics, those with arthritis, diabetes, the blind, the deaf, those who have had bone fractures, traumas of the head, strokes and high blood pressure, the aged, those who have had heart surgery, and many others. More subtle but just as obvious, is the physical and psychological handicap of obesity and overweight that can lead to serious problems.

Aquacise is more than recreation. It is a total body and mind building, goal achieving, creative activity that can benefit everybody in various ways. Water exercises develop and improve all physical capacities of the body while participants are moving in, or are partially submerged in the water. Normal buoyancy of the body relieves the feet and legs of weight. This is especially important for those who have foot, ankle, knee or muscle problems, or who have varicose veins.

Each water exercise program should be divided into three parts: first, the warm-ups at the beginning and the tapering-off at the end of the session. Most of these exercises are similar or may be interchanged. The middle, or the main part of the session is spent in conditioning to strengthen major muscle groups and to stretch and develop flexibility. This is combined with aerobics to improve the circulatory and respiratory systems. For maximum benefits, the sessions should be a half hour in length and from four to five times a week. Two sessions may be scheduled closely together, or taken for three hours weekly. In order to benefit from aquacises or from any other exercise, one must exercise a minimum of twelve minutes continuously at training rate of heartbeat in addition to a warm-up and tapering-off period.

The training rate of the heartbeat is determined by taking the resting heart rate. This should be taken several times in order to know the average. Next, the maximum rate of the heartbeat should be determined by 220 minus your age. This figure should give you the fastest rate your heart should beat for your age. You should not permit yourself to exceed it. Third, you calculate the maximum rate minus your resting rate to give you the training rate that you need to maintain for a minimum of twelve minutes in order to benefit from any exercise.

Even if you are a whiz at arithmetic, you must be safe and secure regarding your maximum and your training rates of heartbeat. Be certain to check all rates with your physician. You may also visit a preventive medical center to take a stress ECG examination. Before and during your participation in an exercise program, take this stress test at least once a year.

If you have ever had any problems with your heart, with blood pressure, with diabetes, with circulation -- or with arithmetic -- be certain to check your figures with your doctor.

In addition to knowing your resting heart rate, your training heart rate, your maximum heart rate, and how to properly take your pulse at your throat, there are some other things you should record before you begin an exercise program.

Without taking a deep breath or sucking in your tummy, honestly record your measurements: waist; hips; right thigh; left thigh; right ankle; left ankle; right leg calf; left leg calf; right upper and lower arm. Measure your chest, and then take the deepest possible breath and measure your chest expansion. Be sure to record your blood pressure.

Finally, you should determine your goals. Do you want to reduce all measurements but the chest expansion, or do you simply want to lose pounds? Maybe you want to gain weight -- solid, not flabby tissue.

If you simply want to lose pounds, forget aquacises, forget jogging, forget cycling, and forget all other forms of exercise that make you fit. You can die comfortably on the golf course, at the bowling alley, at the bridge table, or while you watch your favorite television program. This does not mean that pounds are unimportant; they are, but just losing pounds or just losing fat should not be your fitness goal. Pounds and fat are not the health culprits.

The lack of well trained and conditioned muscle tissue is the villain. As you continue to munch before the idiot box, as you deceive yourself into believing you are getting good exercise as you ride around in a golf cart or drink beer in the local bowling alley, your muscles turn to fat and they degenerate. The chemistry of the muscles that remain change, so that they burn fewer and fewer calories. You become fat. Eventually you are obese.

Fat! An ugly word; so you frantically diet and you join others who compare calories and pounds. You phone friends when you are tempted to eat that goodie, and you become conscious of being an eataholic.

Most dieting is the result of panic and the desire to get slim (or normal) quickly. Actually, diet without exercise (even with exercise) can not help your firmness and fitness because it can not affect our muscle tissue or change the chemistry of the muscles. Unwise dieting can inhibit fitness by the body's consuming not only fat but also healthy muscle tissue.

At first the dieter gets weak for he/she is losing muscle tissue as well as fat. A lumpy and poorly proportioned fat person may become a lumpy and poorly proportioned skinny person. A skinny person may remain obese, have little muscle tissue in proportion to flab or fat. Fat people float wonderfully because fatty tissue cells contain oxygen.

Just as fat (or bones) show, so fitness shows in the toning of the body's muscles and in the improvement of the shape of the torso, legs, arms, and the whole body as a result of developing neglected muscles. Muscles become lean as the marbled fat disappears and is replaced by lean tissue. There is a positive modification within the whole body, for the cumulative effect of exercise is as powerful as the cumulative effect of calories and inactivity.

Exercise increases the metabolic rate and alters the chemistry of muscles and other tissues. The cumulative effect of exercise makes a more efficient furnace of your body, and causes you to burn an increasing number of calories while you ride a golf cart, sit before the boob tube, or even while you sleep. Likewise, after you have been exercising for a few weeks, or a few months, depending upon the individual, your appetite becomes less and your intake of food much less.

I have seen people who were too fat to squeeze between the hand-holds in order to use the steps leading into the swimming pool become truly trim. One woman who lost 175 pounds and got down to 200 pounds, was overjoyed that she could do an increasing number of water exercises and extend the length of her sessions. She not only lost gross fat, she became firm. She does not have dimpled legs or flabby arms, and her flesh doesn't hang like sack cloth from her bones.

This woman's problem was very common: which comes first, the chicken or the egg. Should she lose weight before she exercised, or should she exercise before she lost weight? I advised her to lose some weight with a sensible diet -- without counting calories -- so that exercise would not overly tax her heart or her other organs. I recommended daily aquacises because running, even slow walking, would put great stress on her feet, ankles, legs and back. The water would support her weight so that she could exercise without causing injury to these parts, and she would not unnecessarily risk developing varicose veins. After she had lost enough weight to move with some ease without taxing her heart, she began a serious program of adding other exercises to aquacises.

From the very beginning I told her to modify her diet, not to go on a diet! She cut out all sweets and desserts such as pies, pastries, ice cream, cake and candies -- also salt, potato chips and other junk foods, since even those without salt often contain a lot of fat. I advised her to eliminate all forms of pork, including bacon and ham, all gravies, and to seldom eat starches or potatoes with butter or sour cream. She substituted yams (really a form of squash), salt substitutes, yogurt instead of butter or margarine, and to lower cholesterol she used olive oil, skimmed milk cheeses and cottage cheese. I gave her a list of dietary taboos and another list of necessary foods, including seafood at least four days a week. Next, I told her to make certain that she grocery shopped AFTER she had a satisfying meal, never when she was slightly hungry. I agreed to give her the lists and to advise her only under the condition that she would check everything I said with her doctor and have tests for diabetes, thyroid and other problems. It is much wiser -- and more convenient -- to know the foods you should and should not eat or drink than it is to be a slave to a calorie chart of special dishes. Generally speaking, one needs to modify a whole lifestyle and cooking practices, gradually and sensibly, and to schedule exercises. This has worked for most of the seniors in my water exercise classes. We both felt triumphant when this lady became stable at 160 pounds. More than one doctor had told her it would be impossible for her to ever reach a normal weight. Others had suggested stomach staples and other surgery. Instead we worked on developing a good body -- not on simply losing pounds. I insisted that she trash her swim suit that looked like a tent with a skirt and buy a form revealing leotard type -- bright red. I was afraid she might become so self-conscious that she wouldn't want to be seen in the pool; instead, she hurried into the water which she felt concealed her "rolls." At first she swathed herself in a huge bath towel as she crossed to the pool area. Even though the water is crystal clear she (and other obese people) tend to feel inconspicuous when they are submerged. Wearing a form-fitting swimsuit motivates them to work harder so they'll look acceptable in them.

In this same aquacise class were two men and a woman who'd had extensive heart surgery, two people who'd had strokes, and several who had (now lowered) dangerously high blood pressure. All of these people were handicapped, but they worked hard a minimum of three days a week in half hour aquacise classes. They all now enjoy freedom from fat, freedom of movement, and freedom from thinking they could not solve their physical and psychological problems.

None of these people knew how to swim, and some were very afraid of the water. They overcame their fear -- another freedom. Aquacising makes fitness possible.

Aquacise not only makes it possible for people with distressing handicaps to achieve improved health, but it paves the way for participating in other sports and activities. I am not saying that aquacise is the only way to get fit, but it is the most efficient and pleasurable way to get yourself fit enough to swim, to jog, to walk, to ride horseback, to cycle, to jump rope, or to do any other exercise. Aquacising is more than recreation; it is a total body building program that may be enjoyed in a class with others or alone. It may be practiced in a small or a large pool, in fairly deep or shallow water. It is a sure way of achieving the following objectives.

First, exercising aims at improving or initiating physical fitness in three ways. It develops strength, endurance, and stamina through aerobics and conditioning. It develops or enhances flexibility, agility, and coordination. Aquacising prevents or can cure insomnia. In so doing it eliminates the urge or the necessity to take tranquilizers, sleeping aids, or other drugs. It improves circulation and the heart's efficiency. It cures common constipation, and eliminates the need for laxatives.

The second aim of aquacise is to discourage the use of alcohol and all drugs, mainly because aquacising eliminates most reasons for drinking. Many people drink in order to "turn on" and to sharpen or intensify their emotions or dulled perceptions; however, experiencing positive emotions and a sense of well-being results from the stimulation of good exercise. If one swims, cycles, etc., he has a good "high" without seeking any other source of "kicks." He becomes alert. People often drink in order to relax. After a good exercise session, muscles and all parts of the body and mind are automatically relaxed. Sometimes people drink in order to forget their problems or because they feel sorry for themselves; they seek escape. They long for the good old days, for youth and sparkle. Aquacising may -- or may not -- provide socializing, but it occupies the mind, and self pity is replaced by a special kind of pride. It can not revive the good old days, but it can enrich the present and make life worth living now.

The third aim of aquacises is the development of special pride that can become self-satisfaction, even conceit. Water exercises are associated with many other kinds of psychological benefits. They firm and reduce body dimensions and get rid of rolls and dimples; automatically improving the individual's appearance. This improved appearance improves the self-image through heightened awareness of the physical impression.

The sense of what the body does and how it moves, kinesthetic awareness, is sharpened; thus a person's walk and other movements require less effort. He or she no longer slumps, pants after climbing stairs, or slouches. This improvement in the appearance of the body, in the self-image, and in posture and movement tend to make people want to display themselves and to have contact with others who exercise. Socializing easily becomes another by-product.

The fourth objective of aquacising is the promotion of safety. As a person becomes comfortable in the water he subconsciously learns to breathe and to move in what was once a strange medium. He may not be aware of learning the use of buoyancy, of specific gravity, of balance and his center of gravity, and of how to move in the water. Subconsciously, he learns the nature of the laws of motion in water: the law of stationary and moving inertia; the law of acceleration; the law of action and reaction, and the law of leverage. Repetition of simple exercises teaches him some elementary skills, such as maintainingprone position, gliding, kicking, and even proper breathing in the water.

Other objectives of exercising include relaxation from strain and pressure; arresting of the aging process; making people alert and efficient on their jobs; creating a sense of timing, rhythm, and pure pleasure.

Rhythm, the repetition of similar effects, equal accents or beats, at approximately equal intervals, or the recurrence of a regular beat in a sequence of units, permeates all life and all art. Animals' heartbeats and muscle contractions are rhythmic throughout normal lives. The muscles contract alternately with a period of relaxation and action or tension. Likewise, our skeletal muscles can work for a long time without fatigue if their contractions alternate regularly with complete relaxation. This relaxation provides opportunity for replacement of the blood supply that brings oxygen to repair the effects of contraction and to remove metabolic by-products. The rhythm of work and rest reduces fatigue.

Rhythm is a natural part of life and is typical of skilled movement. It is hard to imagine a dancer or a swimmer who does not have rhythm. Rhythm is the result of forces that include muscular contractions that combine to create movement and to overcome a specific resistance. The proper sequence of the application of these forces creates timing. Duration, the time it takes to perform a movement, and the number of times a movement is repeated are important in performing all exercise. The speed of performance of a movement depends upon its duration. When the duration is decreased, the speed should be increased.

Conditioning and aquacising aim to enhance the properties of the muscles: their extensibility, their elasticity, their contractility, and their amplitude.

Extensibility refers to the muscle fibers' stretchability rather than to the stretchability of the tendons and the ligaments that are not ordinarily extensible. On the other hand, muscle fiber can be stretched one-third to one-half its normal resting length. If muscles are suddenly stretched, these fibers likely will rupture, especially where the junction of the muscle fibers meet the tendon. When capillaries rupture, one usually sees a bruise, and although it may seem that a muscle is repaired after having been abused or stretched suddenly, it never is the same again; it loses its original flexibility. Because of the pressure and the resistance of water, it is not as easy to injure or to overly stretch a muscle in the water as it is in the air. The range through which a muscle can operate from its most completely extended position through elastic recoil and a full concentric contraction, is known as muscle amplitude. Stretch-reflex occurs when a muscle's fiber is

stretched and responds normally by contracting. Improvement of the strength and performance of muscles usually is accomplished by overloading through the use of weights, through changes of body positions, through isometrics, and through tempo. Power is not strength; power results when strength is applied. Power is acquired through coordination and muscle strength, through muscle tone, and through adequate conditioning. Aquacises and swimming will develop long, not bulky or bunchy, muscles.

The basic exercises in this book are aimed at activating all parts of the body and strengthening the muscles in order to create and preserve fitness. These exercises are not designed for working the parts of your body independently. There is no specific exercise for your big toe or for your right eyebrow because every exercise contributes to the strengthening and conditioning of your whole body. Of course, some movements do emphasize neck, back, or hip flexibility.

Bent leg lifts, for example, obviously tighten stomach and lower back muscles, but they also strengthen legs, hips and waist.

Aquacises are simple; yet you should try to perfect each one with practice. Begin with relatively easy exercises and gradually add the more difficult ones. Begin by repeating each exercise from five to ten times during each session. The speed used in executing movements will, and should, increase with practice.

The only way to derive full benefit from these exercises is to do them every day. If it is sometimes impossible to do them in the water, do them wherever you happen to be, in or out of water, but do them. Whenever possible, exercise before meals.

Select several exercises from each section of this book for your daily sessions. You do not need or want to perform all the warm-ups and taper-offs in one session. You should, however, select several of these as well as several conditioning and aerobic exercises. The sample aquacise short session in the appendix of this book may be a helpful guide. It is important to plan your sessions to include all three kinds of exercises. Your body needs the variety.

If at first you fail to execute an exercise, then try to do it until you can perform it with ease. Do not hurry. Do not injure a muscle by suddenly stretching it beyond your comfortable limits; however, take care to do the exercise correctly, even if you do not entirely achieve it. The instructor's positions are calculated to give maximum benefits. For example, if you can not touch your nose to your knee on the ballet barre leg stretch (done on the pool gutter), be certain to keep both legs straight and continue to bend towards the knee. Keep the hips parallel to the pool wall and do not twist your body in order to lower your head.

Wear a simple, leotard type swim suit that does not pull between the shoulders or at the crotch. The suit should fit snugly. Beware of straps that slip and must be constantly "hiked" over the shoulder. If the suit is figure revealing -- O.K.; you will work to look well in it. If you don't wear a bathing cap, be sure to tie back your hair so it won't fall across your face and inhibit your movements. You may need to wear swimming goggles if you have sensitive eyes or if you swim after exercising.

At first do stretches slowly, gradually increasing your speed. Never sacrifice form for speed. Remember, in order to benefit from aquacise or almost any other exercise, it is necessary to exercise continuously for twelve minutes at training heart rate in addition to warming up and tapering off.

Happy fitness! Happy aquacising!

WARM-UPS AND
TAPER-OFFS

The beginning and ending exercises of your session may be exchanged. The warm-upper period should last five minutes. The taper-off period should also last a good five minutes. Exercise at a moderate rate and do *not* reach your target heart level. Walking and running through waist-deep water is always good. Select exercises that use all major muscle groups. Movements should be slow and relaxed. Try twists, side bends, walking variations, kickboard exercises.

Most exercises are a bit more strenuous in shallow water. Your heart rate should slow to 100 or lower at the end of the cool down section. If your pulse has not adequately lowered, move slowly in the water until it does come down.

Before you create anything there are certain things you need to do in order to ensure pleasurable and effective procedure. Any carpenter can tell you the importance of having the proper tools and plans on hand. An artist needs his stretched canvas, his charcoal, his paints and his time budgeted. A writer needs to master mechanics of sentence structure, punctuation and various forms of composition. He needs rich and living experience and he needs his typewriter or word-processor. A cook needs the utensils, the groceries and the recipe.

You need to take some special steps if you want to develop a stronger and more attractive body as well as an improved personality and sense of well-being. Health and success are not accidents or simply the result of luck. They are the result of dedicated work and self-discipline. You create your own fitness.

According to the U.S. President's Council on Physical Fitness and Sports, fitness is "the ability to carry out daily tasks efficiently with enough energy left over to enjoy leisure time pursuits and to meet unforeseen emergencies."

Even though fitness is a relative thing that is partly determined by your physiological composition, your general health, your age, sex, your body type, your life style, etc.; even more, it is a psychological thing. Only you can decide how fit you want to be. You should do a little reading on the components of fitness and its six factors: body composition (your body shape and proportions plus your weight to size ratio); your flexibility (the range of movements of each joint that is determined by the mobility of your muscles, tendons and ligaments); your body efficiency (amount of energy you get from a set amount of energy you take in as food); your muscular strength (maximum force a muscle or muscle group can apply in one contraction); muscular endurance (length of time special muscles can continue to perform a special task and the number of repetitions of a movement or a sequence), and finally, cardio-muscular (CR) fitness, or how well your heart and lungs can supply the active muscles with oxygen and remove the waste products.

As one gets older it seems as if all these components degenerate, but that does not necessarily have to be true. Naturally, some components may become less efficient than others, for example, a person with arthritis loses flexibility of joints; yet he can compensate for some of this by emphasizing muscular strength and endurance. Diabetics not only have to emphasize maintaining their normal body composition and CR fitness, but they have to daily monitor their blood content and provide for intelligent use of energy. This is true for diabetics of all ages. It is necessary that they structure and schedule their lives. Both Type I and Type II diabetics have to carefully monitor their body efficiency.

Whether we are five or fifty there is not a lot we can do about our body composition. Some people are (fat) endomorphic; some are (muscular) mesomorphic, and others are (thin) ectomorphic. If one is endomorphic, he should realize that his type has more frequent coronary problems than the other types. The endomorphics need to give special attention to diet, overexercising, and other factors, but the endomorphic cannot become the "long stemmed American beauty" type regardless of how hard she works at it. I was born a square mesomorphic body type, often referred to as a fire hydrant, and nothing can change that -- when I was sixteen or while I am in my late sixties. On the other hand, I find that I can not do cartwheels around the block or touch my toe to the back of my head as easily as I once did.

Especially senior citizens must be conscious of cardio-vascular and respiratory (CR) fitness as the primary factor in overall physical fitness at all ages. Even arthritis victims (young and old) must work on maintaining their ranges of motion. Other factors include your motor abilities, your coordination, agility, balance, speed of movement, reaction time, and power. As we age we lose some of each of these. Aquacise helps prevent uncomfortable -- sometimes tragic -- loss of all of them.

Unfortunately,most people know more about their car's engine or their washing machines than they know about their own bodies. So you can go to a repairman -- or a doctor. Most people speak more intelligently with salesmen of homes, of cars, of appliances, and with brokers than they do with their doctors about their own bodies. Your physician and your dentist can be of much greater help to you if you have a little background knowledge about your body and your mind. You can trade in your car, but this is the only body you will have -- in this lifetime. Prepare yourself by knowing some basic things about yourself.

Start by keeping a large calendar, notebook or diary -- all about you. Begin by taking your weight, your measurements, and your chest expansion. Be sure to measure your upper and lower arms, the calves of your legs and your thighs, your neck and your ankles. You will later be surprised when you again take your measurements and discover that you have lost inches -- and maybe you have gained weight. Honestly look at your-self, naked and from all angles, in a full length mirror. Periodically do this, and you will be pleased to see the "sacks" disappear, the dimples go and a gradual change to sculptured, smooth, long lines created by those long muscles under firm flesh. Keep an accurate record of your heart rate: rate at rest, training rate, and moderate movement rates.

Do not start an aquacise program or any other exer-cise program until you have seen your physician and he has given his approval. Your doctor should know you and your body; he should know your present capacity to perform specific exercise, and he should know your potential. His approval and his advice should always precede your starting to do any exercise. Very likely he has suggested long ago that you exercise. If you do not have a serious physical problem, he should have sug-gested it.

On the other hand, once when I was new in an area I consulted a well known physician who insisted that I take it very easy and if I moved at all I should stroll, not even walk fast. I immediately distrusted him and got a "second opinion." My present physician believes in two things mainly: salads and exercise.

Often people are not critical enough to get second opinions or to see more than one physician. Others ignore a good physician's advice to stop smoking, not to drink, to eat sensibly, and to exercise. A good doctor wants to be part of a team in helping you develop healthy and happy living. One criteria for trusting a doctor is his emphasis upon preventive medicine rather than having you stuff your purse or pocket with prescriptions. His success is not counted in caskets.

After you have the approval of your doctor to begin an Aquacise Program, locate a convenient, clean and safe pool. People from Seattle and Washington's King County are fortunate to have their Forward Thrust Swimming Pools, many of which have "Swim and Trim," water exercise programs. Des Moines, Washington's Mt. Rainier Pool has four levels of water exercise programs: Swim.and Trim for a half hour of exercises for average people; Water Aerobics for one hour for those who are young and fit; Senior Exercises for people over fifty, and Arthritis Exercises for those with arthritis or other severe physical problems. All four classes are offered a minimum of three times a week throughout the year. Not every city or county has numerous swimming pools with trained staff; however, you should phone your local county Parks and Recreation Department to learn what is offered. If there is no aquatic program or no available public pool, try to find a private one, maybe an apartment or condo complex with a pool.

Now you have a copy of *Aquacises,* your physician's directions and his approval, and you have located a pool and have its schedule. You have a notebook with your measurements, your heart rates, and other special and personal data.

You have not quite completed your preparations. Jot down in the intimate notebook some practical and immediate objectives for yourself. "I want to lose an inch around my waist before Easter (or Passover)." "I aim to be able to swim a hundred yards without stopping in a month." Do not make your objectives impossible or too numerous. Save the big suckers for someplace near the back of the book: "I aim to wear size __ and not have flat feet by Christmas." You may reach that big objective by the time all the pages are filled.

Meanwhile, get your gear together. Start by getting a swim suit. Do not wear shorts and a sweat shirt even though you think that they camouflage your spare tires and bulges. Be dangerous. Be bold. Get a one piece Speedo, Head, or Arena suit that exposes your figure problems. The more a suit demands a sleek body, the harder you will work and the more improvement you will make. You might feel more comfortable by sticking to blacks and blues, but reds will make you want to firm up faster. Avoid department stores' sales of skirted and fashionable "tents." Fashion suits often have arm holes that are so small they chafe you or inhibit movements. Most of them are poorly designed for anything but beach sunning. Avoid lycra and stick to nylon. Lycra stretches badly and thus gives you a false sense of accomplishment as you think you are shrinking, when actually the suit is stretching,

You may want a swim cap. Beginning swimmers usually have dry hair or wear those fancy hats with rubber flowers. Some people even wear shower caps. What you need is a tight, simple Speedo cap, often worn with the ears exposed since water stays in the ears if a cap is worn over them. Do not use a cap with a chin strap; the strap can cut off circulation or inhibit proper breathing. Forget about trying to keep your hair dry; that is not the purpose of a cap. The purpose of the cap is to prevent your hair from draping over your eyes or from swishing through the water. If you are in the water daily, be sure to shower out the pool water and chlorine, but do not shampoo daily. Simply rinse well and finish off with a good conditioner. Too much shampoo will dry your hair. Hair length does not matter; mine is waist long and wet daily, but my style is so simple that I do not take any time for it. I avoid using a hairdryer unless it is absolutely necessary. My hair usually is dry sooner than those who fool around under dryers. Often I wear no hat but braid my hair or tie it into a pony tail. Check pool rules; some places require patrons to wear caps. Serious swimmers are seldom style-conscious. They often wear old and faded suits; when suits become thin, they wear two suits.

Until you are an accomplished diver do not invest in a mask or snorkel -- ever! They inhibit proper breathing and a mask can actually be very dangerous. They never should be used by children; in fact, it should be against the law to sell them to the general public. Unless you are a synchronized swimmer, never wear nose clips or plugs. Never wear ear plugs; they hold water in the ear. Normally, the only things you should wear are a swim suit and simple cap. If you have foot problems or if you are a beginner with fins, wear white socks. Socks can protect your feet from the cement pool bottom, or prevent blisters under fins.

If you have eye problems or if your eyes are exposed under water for a long period, wear goggles. Get clear ones for indoor pools, and use colored ones only for outdoor pools to protect your eyes from surface glare or from the sun.

Decent pools require all bathers to shower (soap showers in Canada) before they enter the pool. Take a nice, warm shower -- get the suit and cap wet -- before you go to the pool. The pool water will feel great, but if you do not shower, your body may feel an unpleasant shock from the chilly water. Everyone's showering keeps the PH down in the pool. When you leave the pool, *DO NOT TAKE A HOT SHOWER*; a tepid or cool shower will be fine.

Never smoke in or around an athletic complex of any kind. Smoke is very bad for people who do deep breathing and it can be very dangerous in the vicinity of chlorine. Never chew gum or keep it in your mouth. You could choke on it very easily.

Unless you are in an exercise class that is directed by a trained instructor, take your lesson plan with you. Until you are practiced you likely will forget the exercises you want to do. It is a good idea to make three plans for three days of the week so that you can get both practice and variety. At the back of this text is a sample plan that includes the three main parts: warm-ups, conditioning and aerobics, and taper-offs. Try to make your plans so that you work-out a minimum of a half hour plus ten minutes of warm-ups and five to ten minutes of taper-offs. Balance your plan by selecting exercises from each of the parts of this book. Write your plan on sturdy paper in pencil only; ink runs. When you enter the pool, simply dip the paper lightly into the water; then spread it near the edge of the pool where you will be exercising. Dampness will prevent its blowing away or being misplaced; yet it will be close enough for you to read.

If the pool does not have a pace clock, use an inexpensive water resistant watch (there is no such thing as a completely waterproof watch) that is easily read. Be sure to remove the lesson plan when you finish so you will not litter the pool.

Beside your lesson plan place all the equipment you may need, such as a kickboard, wrist weights, arm or leg floaters, pull buoys, etc. Even though you may not need everything you put there, if you change your mind and decide you need something, it is distressing and time wasting to have to leave the pool to get equipment. If you have time left over after your exercise session, repeat some exercises or walk or run in the pool if you cannot swim. Begin slowly with less strenuous exercises; as you gain experience put in longer sessions with more intense or faster exercises. Keep your movements smooth and fluid, never stiff or jerky. Pause periodically and take your pulse to see if you are over or under your training rate.

Warm-up exercises prevent a shock to your body. One of the best ways to warm-up is to walk and then run back and forth across the shallow end of the pool. Some people like to sit on the side of the pool and do simple out of the water exercises before going in. This slowly increases the flow of blood to your capillaries. Before you entered the water, your muscles were comparatively at rest and had a minimum of blood supply. As you gradually increase the tempo of your work, muscles require a full and constant blood supply; you are simply feeding your body in preparation for more strenuous activity.

Your heart is the most important muscle in your body, and the heart, like the other muscles, is twenty percent more elastic and more efficient when it is warm. Likewise, if you are careful to warm up your body, you will run less risk of pulling muscles, and your whole body will be less vulnerable to aches, cramps, or worse. Periodically check your pulse to see if your heart rate is approaching the proper training rate.

Warm-up exercises may be more important for swimmers and for those who exercise in the water than for joggers or others who exercise on land simply because the body temperature drops immediately upon entering the water. You must work to move that blood through your body. When you become accustomed to aquacising, your skin should be flushed pink when you finish your conditioning and aerobics.

Just as you should run your automobile engine a few minutes before you drive, and just as you should walk a horse before you ride it, so you should warm up your own body before you do heavy exercises.

On the other hand, you should always taper off your exercise period. When you suddenly stop exercising, your heart continues to pump at a rapid rate for a while. Your heart just does not know that you are quitting for the day, and it will continue to pump an excessive amount of blood that collects temporarily in your veins and muscles. This can cause you to chill or to feel dizzy or light-headed. Your taper-off exercises get your body accustomed, again, to less activity. This gives your circulatory system as well as your muscles the opportunity to safely adapt to another pace.

There are authorities who believe that it is downright dangerous not to warm up or to taper off if doing heavy exercising, and no exercise is really worth doing unless it is done hard, done well, and done appropriately. You should take as long to taper off as you do to warm up, a minimum of five minutes for middle aged people and ten minutes for senior citizens. Make certain that your recovery heart rate is less than 120 beats per minute. Ten minutes after you completely stop exercising or get out of the water, your breathing rate should be normal and comfortable, about twelve to sixteen breaths per minute. Your five minute recovery heart-beat rate should be less than 120 beats per minute. If you continue to breathe hard for longer than that or if the heart rate is not down to 120, it's likely you worked too hard or you may possibly have some type of lung or respiratory problem.

Safety is imperative. Be alert for immediate signs of overexertion during your exercise session. Watch for these warning signs:

1. Any pain in the chest

2. Lightheadedness and/or dizziness

3. Loss of muscle control

4. General or intense weakness

5. Nausea or vomiting after exercising

6. Overly fatigued; drowsiness in later part of the day or fitful tossing and insomnia at night.

If you should experience any of these symptoms, immediately cease exercising. If checking with your physician indicates that your condition is normal, reduce the intensity or the duration of your activity. Whenever such a symptom continues, get medical attention.

Just as you do not want your heart to pump too much blood after you cease exercising, neither should you suddenly stop moving or exercising and increase warmth. The blood pools and the surface capillary vessels dilate keeping a great percentage of blood away from the heart. Therefore, never take a hot shower or go into a sauna or steam room immediately after exercising.

On the other hand, a cold shower or cold temperatures can cause leg cramps and be a bad shock to the body. Use moderation in such circumstances and take only a slightly warm or tepid shower. This is very important for young children and senior citizens.

Some people advocate wearing shorts and letting the body cool while one walks rapidly or runs. The contrast of your warm body and the cool air can also be a shock to the body; so I advocate wearing full length sweats during and for a while after exercising. Unless the weather is very tropical, wear sweats when you leave (and enter) the pool locker rooms. Even in Florida and Alabama summers, the ballet groups with whom I danced wore leotards, tights, and knitted leg warmers during work-outs and for our cooling off periods. We didn't take cold showers -- or hot ones.

Now you are warmed up and your muscles have increased their elasticity, your veins and arteries have opened up pathways to the muscles you will use, and your body temperature has risen to help facilitate bio-chemical reactions that will feed energy to your muscles' tissues. ENJOY!

PRE-PLUNGERS

After you have showered and are ready to enter the water, it is a good idea to sit on the edge of the pool and do a few warm-up, out of the water movements. If you are a confirmed toe-toucher, be cautious never to bounce up and down. Do not bounce these suggested exercises but maintain a moderate and smooth transition between positions or movements. Sit far enough back on the edge of the pool so that you do not tumble into the water head first. Be cautious of slick edges.

1. Sit so that your legs hang over the edge of the pool -- legs slightly spread apart. Touch each elbow to the opposite knee several times.

2. Sit so that your legs, spread slightly apart, hang over the edge of the pool. Hunch your shoulders and keep your relaxed but straight arms together. Sit erect and then lower your hands towards your feet. At a moderate rate alternate between sitting erect and lowering your arms and hands between your legs.

3. Sit at the side of the pool with your legs reasonably far from the edge so that you will not fall into the water. Spread your legs apart but keep them straight. Bend

from the hips and touch each hand to the
opposite toe or ankle.

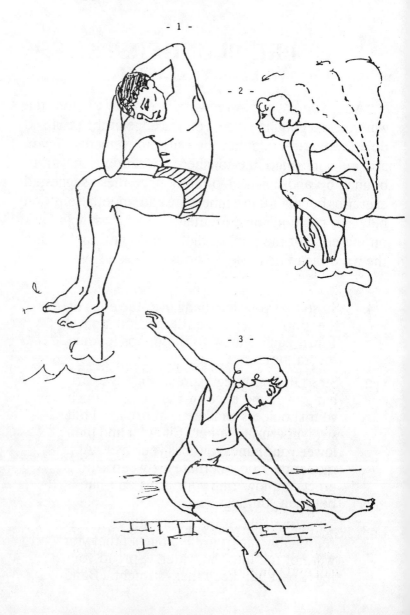

WATER WALKS

Water jogging or stepping can be good for starting and finishing your aquacise sessions. In addition to simple jogging through the water, the following walks are excellent. These should be done in a minimum of waist deep water in order to benefit from the water's resistance. Try doing them across the pool.

1. **The Goose Step:** Place your hands on your hips and stand erect. First lift one straight leg to the surface of the water and then lift the other one. Throughout this walk both legs should be kept perfectly straight. It is important not to bend the body forward or backward and to look straight ahead.

2. **Ribbon Step:** Weave your feet and legs as you move sideways through the water. First one foot and then the other foot crosses in front. Hold the arms out straight and above the water.

3. **Side Step:** As in the Ribbon Step, you keep your side towards the opposite pool wall and you move sideways. Simply pull

your feet and legs together and then separate them using a slight jump.

4. **Hopping:** First bend your right knee and hold your right ankle close to your buttocks with your right hand while you hop across the pool on your left leg. Reverse, and hop on your right leg while you secure your left ankle with your left hand. Finally, hop violently and fast on both feet for another couple of widths.

5. **Jog 1:** Jog like the man in the illustration on Page 36, with your knees brought up high in front, a kind of prancing.

6. **Jog 2:** Jog like the lady, Page 36; keep the knees parallel and bring one foot at a time up to your buttocks.

7. **Stand in Place Swing:** (profile illustration, Page 36) and bring up one knee, foot hanging downward. Swing the foot up to the water's surface; then kick it down again as you keep your knee bent. For variety, swing the lower leg in circles, first several times in one direction and then several times in the opposite direction. Repeat the movements with the other leg.

Explanation

If a group is exercising, the leader can form large circles and use any or all of these water walks. First one group should be directed to go forward as fast as possible, and the leader should unpredictably shout the order to move backwards. The forward/backward instructions should be frequent so that there is greater benefit from water resistance, Even better, those who do the walks should hold kickboards at least three-fourths under water and push them against the current in front -- with straight arms. Reversals will give an obvious push-pull effect with the kickboards. Likewise, it is fun to hop, feet and legs together (Bunny Hop) back and forth over the bottom line markings of the pool. This may be done by using one or both feet, by keeping the body straight or by twisting the body. It may be done forward and backward over the line or from one side of the pool to the other.

Be imaginative and create your own walks and steps. You can try disco-dancing, waltzing, or polkas in the water. You can do these individually or with a partner, with or without music.

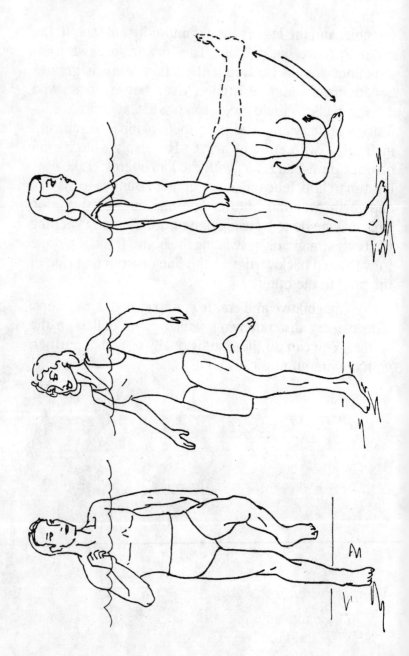

HEAD ROLLERS

Starting Position

These exercises may be done either standing straight or in sitting position. Do not move any part of the body but the head and neck.

Movements

1. Relax, head forward and chin on chest.

2. Slowly look over the right shoulder; then recover.

3. Slowly turn head to the left -- chin to left shoulder. Drop the chin as you again move the head toward right shoulder.

4. Begin by looking straight forward with head in normal and relaxed position. Push the whole head (maybe lead with the chin) forward. Return to starting position.

5. Push the whole head back. Pull in the chin and tighten the muscles at the back of your neck.

Explanation and Caution

These movements should be made slowly and easily. NEVER jerk and NEVER roll the head backward as in illustrations marked X. This exercise is divided so that the head moves in four specific directions: forward, backward (Rubber Necks), and side to side.

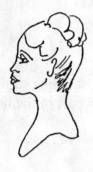

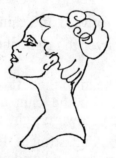

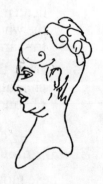

Rubber Necks

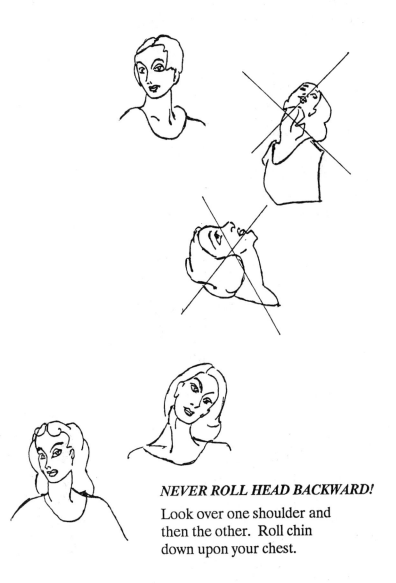

NEVER ROLL HEAD BACKWARD!

Look over one shoulder and
then the other. Roll chin
down upon your chest.

WATERPUSH

Starting Position

With back straight, squat or stand so that the water covers your shoulders. Your arms are extended and stretched out in opposite directions.

Movement

1. Moving from the waist only, keep your arms in opposite directions, and push the water as far right as possible.

2. Then slowly twist and push the water in the opposite direction. You may twist your wrist and form paddles of your hands (fingers closed and palms out).

Explanation

The arms must be kept underwater and straight. Twist the wrists so that you move the water in sweeping motion.

STARTER STRETCH

Starting Position

Stand straight with arms outstretched in opposite directions along the gutter or pool top. Throughout the exercise be sure you keep your whole back, from shoulders to seat, against the side of the pool. The man in the illustration has let his seat move from the side, as do most beginners; try to avoid this.

Movements

1. Slowly bend both knees at the same time and lift them closely to the body and towards the chest.

2. Pretend you are on an invisible swing and pump or bicycle your legs out straight and down in a circular motion.

3. Pull your bent legs so your toes come close to the side of the pool, do not let your toes touch pool bottom.

4. Bicycle both legs together at least ten times.

5. Now reverse the bicycle movement so that you push your toes upward toward the surface.

Variations

Stand on one leg and bicycle the other leg at least ten times; then reverse the cycling movement.

Reverse the legs so that you cycle the other leg the same way. Maintain the position with the body flat against the wall and lift both legs and execute a frog kick. Keep this position and lift the legs; spread them apart and then bring them together, keeping them straight.

First you turn your toes inward so that your toes touch. Then flatten your feet so that your heels (only) meet and separate and then meet again. This is good for the inner thighs.This whole set of exercises is excellent for strengthening and trimming the stomach, the hips and the thighs. Do not try to break the surface of the water with your feet while you do these exercises. Simply keep your legs low -- no higher than the hips.

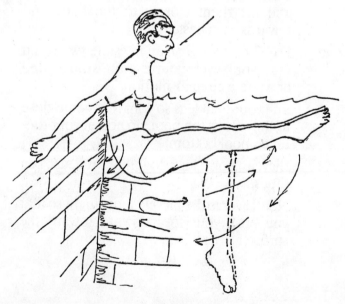

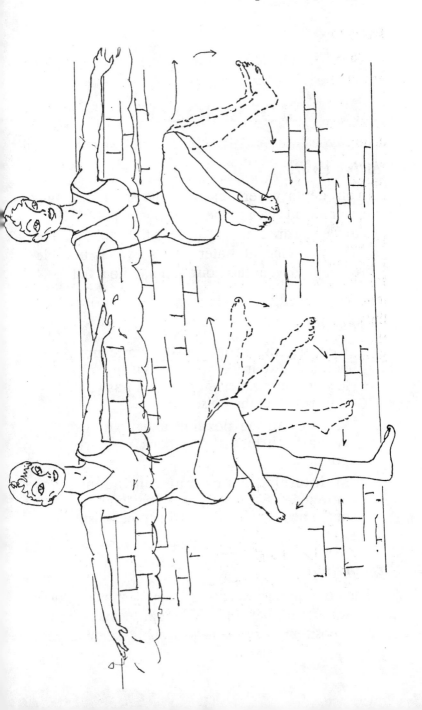

ROLLING LOG

Starting Position

In any depth water, relax and lie on your tummy with your head facing the side of the pool. From head to toe you are at a right angle to the poolside. You may keep your chin at water level so you'll be able to breathe with your face out. Aim to float flat.

Movements

1. Keeping the prone position and not permitting your feet to lower, swing both legs to the right side of the pool as you slowly twist at the waist.

2. Keeping prone position and floating, swing both legs slowly back to start position.

3. Maintaining a slow but continuous movement, swing both legs to the left side of the pool as you slowly twist at the waist.

Explanation

The point of this exercise is to get to moving slowly in the water; so relax and be certain to maintain the floating position. If you have trouble keeping your complete body on the surface of the water with your arms outstretched, try to position one hand at the top of the gutter and keeping the other arm straight, place that hand about two feet directly below the one at the top of the gutter.   Be sure that the hands are in alignment at the center of your body.

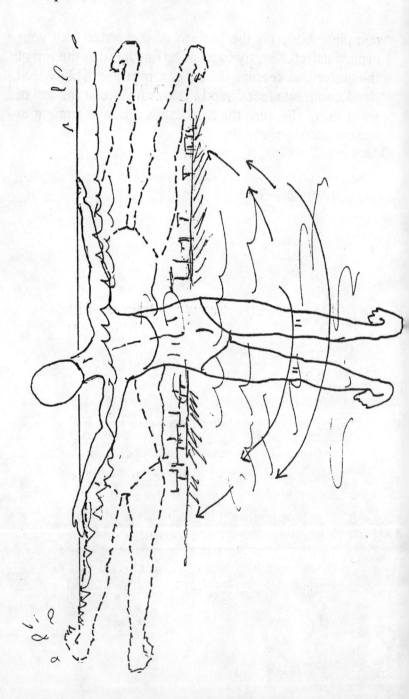

PENDULUM

Starting Position

Stand straight with your whole back, shoulders to seat, against the poolside. Stretch out your arms in opposite directions along the gutter or the side. Legs are together.

Movements

1. Keep both legs straight at all times. Lift the right leg and swing it upward and across your body to your left side so that the right toe touches the pool wall on your left.

2. Without letting your leg drop to the bottom of the pool, and keeping both legs straight, swing the right leg so that your toe touches the pool wall on your right.

3. Repeat movements one and two at least five times.

4. Stand on the right leg and and lift the left leg. Swing the left leg upward and across your body to the left side of the pool. In other words, reverse the exercise and repeat at least five times.

Variation

Stand on one leg and keeping the working leg near the water's surface without letting it drop to the bottom, swing it in a very large figure 8 movement, first to the right and then to the left. Reverse working legs and repeat the movements.

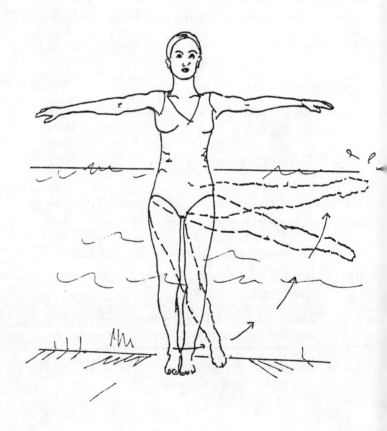

APLAUSE

Starting Position

Stand in shoulder deep water. Be sure to keep your arms and shoulders under the water as you execute this exercise.

Movements

1. Keep your upper arms and elbows close to your sides and quickly clap your hands.

2. Still keeping your arms and your elbows close to your sides, enlarge your movements so that your hands are parallel to and beyond your sides when they are open or apart.

Explanation

The value of this exercise comes from moving against the force of the water. Applaud with the small movement for at least thirty seconds and then applaud with wide movements for about fifteen seconds.

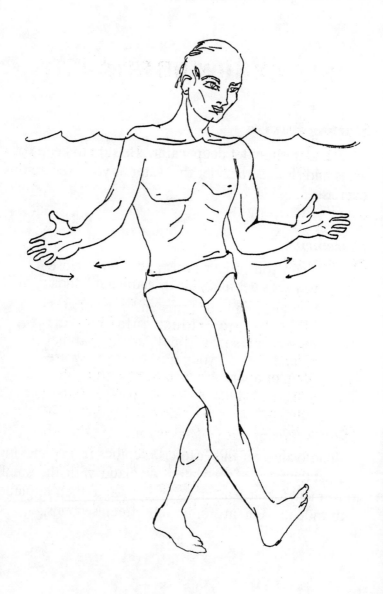

STANDING SIDE STRETCH

Starting Position

Stand in either waist or shoulder deep water. Hands are on your hips. Spread your legs into a wide V, toes pointed bat-footed, in opposite directions, or in a wide ballet second position.

Movements

1. Straighten the right leg and shift your weight so that your left knee is bent over your left toe. Press into this position, your hips turned outward. Keep the torso straight and your chin up.

2. Shift your weight so that you straighten your left leg and shift your weight so that your right knee is bent over the right toe.

3. Keeping your body erect and your hands on your hips or clasped tightly over your head, continue to alternately swing right and left, straightening and bending alternate legs ten times on each side.

Explanation

You should remain in the same spot as you do this exercise. Your feet never move from their initial position. Be sure to turn out your hips and your toes as far as you can. Do this exercise slowly and then rapidly. For variety, throw your arms outward and upward or clasp your hands high above your head as you shift your weight from one foot to the other. Keep your heels on the bottom at all times. For variety, hold a large ball or a kickboard in both hands (arms straight) and bend at the waist so that your arms pull over the side of the bent knee. Also, place your straight arms between your spread legs; bend the elbows and place your head against the side of the pool. Hold the position for a minimum of five seconds; this is a groin stretcher. Of course, your feet have been placed near the top of the sides of the pool, and you hold the pool gutter with your hands.

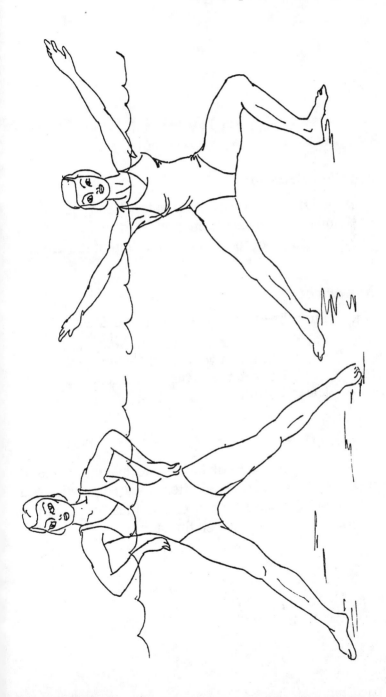

ELBOW PULLS

Starting Position

Stand straight in waist deep water. Bend your elbows at shoulder high level. Clench your fists in front of your chest. Be sure not to drop the elevation of the arms.

Movements

1. Push the elbows back hard three times.
2. On the next push, straighten your arms and try to touch your hands behind your back. Repeat these two movements at least five times.

Explanation

At first you may not be able to make your hands meet behind you; however, after repeated practice your hands will get closer. The exercise must be done very rapidly with your chest well thrust out.

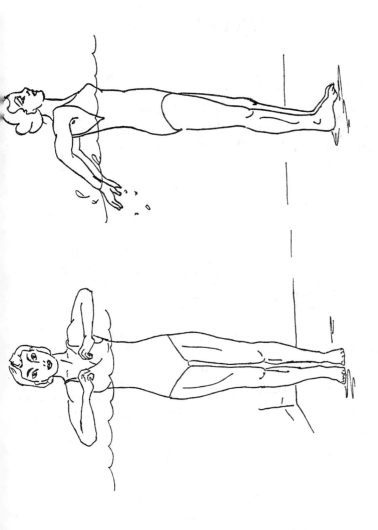

GEOMETRICAL ARMS

Starting Position

Stand in at least waist deep water. Hold up your hands as if someone pointed a gun and said, "Hands up." Bend your elbows after you have extended your arms from the shoulders so that your hands point to the ceiling.

Movements

1. Pivot your forearms (only) and your flattened hands so that they move downward at the same time. Now the fingertips point to the ground.

2. Pivot your forearms (only) and your flattened hands so that they point upward. Your fingertips point towards the ceiling.

3. Straighten both arms in opposite directions; then swing them so that they cross in front of you. The palms of your hands are flat and face downward. Repeat this crossing motion, alternating the top arm.

4. Arms are back into starting position, elbows bent, fingers pointed upward. Repeat the whole cycle of movements rapidly at least ten times.

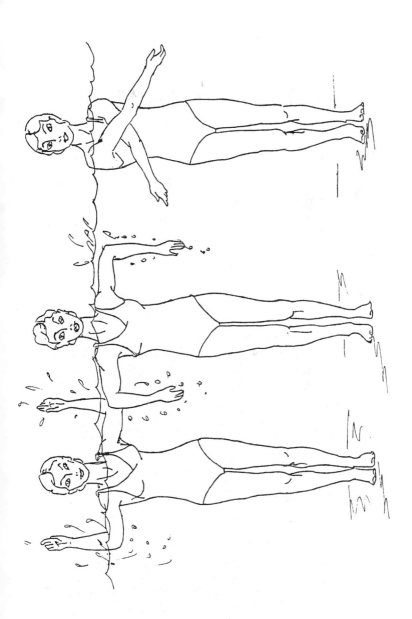

HAND CLUTCHES

Starting Position

Stand in waist deep water with your arms extended straight out in opposite directions. It is preferable to keep the arms underwater; however, the arms may be surfaced. This may also be done in shoulder depth water.

Movements

1. Quickly twist your arms (from the shoulder to the fingertips) forward then backward. At the same time alternate clenching your fists and spreading your fingers.

2. Quickly twist your arms (from the shoulder to the fingertips) backward without lowering your arms. At the same time clench your fists and then open your fingers and stretch them.

Explanation

The twisting of the arms and the clenching and the opening of the fists should be done very rapidly. Do not lower either arm until after you have repeated the exercise several times. It also is a good exercise to simply stand with outstretched arms for a minimum of two to three minutes. For variety hold arms straight up above the head for three or more minutes.

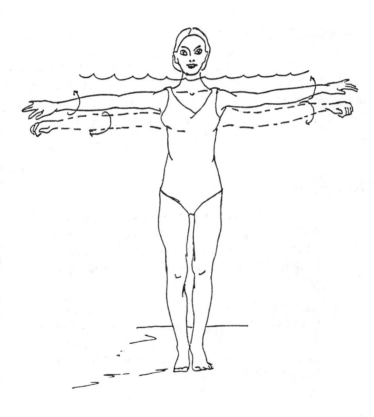

DEMI-PLIES

This is an adaptation of ballet demi-plies (small bendings) and releves (risings).

Starting Position

Stand erect facing the pool wall (so you can balance yourself). Point your toes in opposite directions with your heels together. Turn out your hips and feet, parallel to the wall.

Movements

1. Keep your heels on the ground as you bend your knees directly over your toes. Bend your knees slowly and keep your seat directly under you. Carry your weight on the outer edges of your feet; do not let them roll in on the inside arches.

2. Straighten your legs to starting position.

3. Rise on the balls of your feet as you keep your legs very straight; then return to the starting position with the feet flat. Repeat the whole set of movements a minimum of five times.

Explanation

Rising on the tip-toes or the balls of the feet is called *releve*. This is a ballet *barre* exercise. You miss the point if you are not very careful to turn out your hips as well as your feet. Be sure not to roll your weight to the inner or the arch part of your feet. Not only can this exercise help posture and knees but it is excellent for helping to strengthen the arches of the feet. Do not do this exercise if you have a hip replacement or hip problems. If it is done in the water it is harmless to the knees.

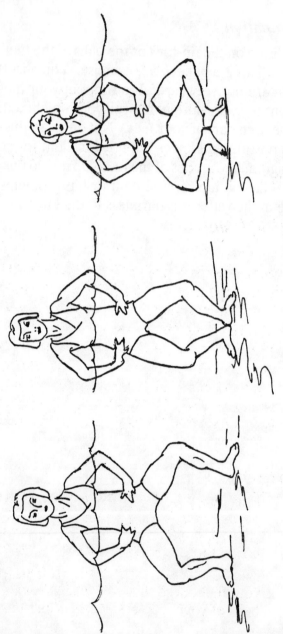

Demi-Plies and Grand Plies

GRAND PLIES

This is an adaptation of ballet's grand plies (large bends) with the releve.

Starting Positions

Stand erect facing the pool wall, using the gutter to balance yourself as you did in executing *demi-plies*. Point your toes in opposite directions with your heels touching. Turn out your hips, parallel to the wall. This should be done in waist deep water. As your skill improves, you may want to do this exercise away from the wall. In which case, you may extend your arms over the surface of the water or put your hands on your hips. Both *grand plies* and *demi-plies* may be done by using any or all of the five standard ballet foot positions illustrated.

Movements

1. Keep your heels on the ground as you begin to bend your knees directly over your toes. Keep your back straight and do not tilt your body forward or backward.

2. As you squat as deeply as possible, roll your feet out so that your weight is on the balls of your feet, or *demi-toe* (half toe).

Keep your back straight and your hips, knees, and toes turned out.

3. Slowly straighten your legs until you are standing in starting position, heels together.

4. *Releve* (rise) slowly from flat-footed position to tip-toes (*releve* position) a few seconds before you lower your heels.

Explanation

I suggest that you do the *grand plies* after you have done the *demi-plies*. Both should be done very slowly. You get a lot of stretch value from the exercises; however, the top thigh muscles may cramp at first and be stiff the next day. Beginners should execute at least three slow plies and then at least four fast ones. Actually, the plies should be done in each of the five ballet foot positions. Each position is kept throughout the series of movements of both exercises. People with hip replacements, hip problems or serious knee problems should avoid *grand plies*.

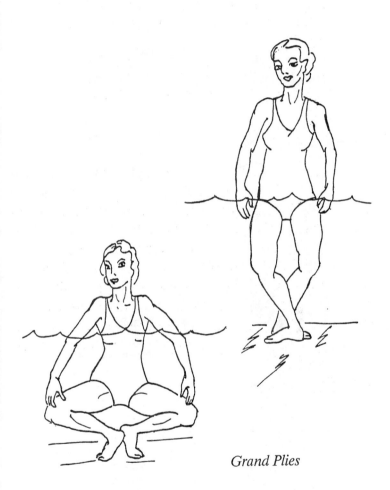

Grand Plies

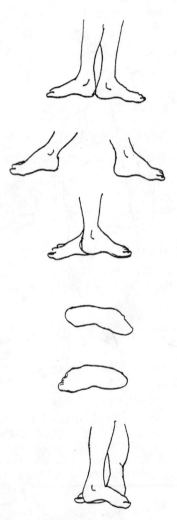

First Position

Heels together, toes in opposite directions

Second Position

As in first, but feet spread parallel

Third Position

Heel of front foot touches arch of back foot

Fourth Position

Feet pointed in opposite directions; one foot placed in front of other foot

Fifth Position

Feet turned outward with toes and heels pointed in exactly opposite directions

FIVE STANDARD BALLET FOOT POSITIONS

TIP-TOES

Starting Position

Stand erect and clasp your hands behind your head. Raise your elbows as high as you can without bringing them forward or backward.

Movements

1. Raise your heels off the bottom of the pool and stand on your tip-toes. Keep your hands clasped behind your neck or head.

2. Return to initial position, feet flat and arms to the sides.

3. Again, clasp your hands behind your neck or your head and rise on your tip-toes. Raise the elbows and walk in very small circles without looking down. Repeat the exercise about seven times.

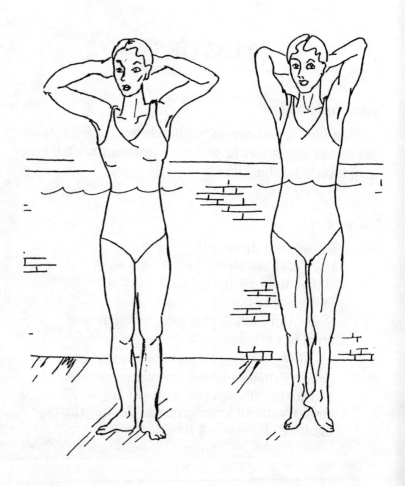

PUSH-AWAYS

Starting Position

For both versions of this exercise stand straight, hands in front of your body, elbows slightly bent. Stand at least a step away from the wall. Either face the wall or have your side to the wall in chest deep water.

Movements

1. Keeping your legs straight and your feet flat with heels on bottom, shift your weight forward toward the wall. Use your hands as buffers and push your body away from the wall to a vertical position again. Repeat this at least ten times.

2. Stand with your side to the wall and fall against your hand that is on the wall. Keep your body straight and your heels on the bottom of the pool. One arm hangs relaxed beside your body; the other arm is bent. Do the exercises ten times on each side.

Variations

Resume starting position; then modify it by placing your heels at the angle where the pool bottom meets the pool wall. Place your toes up against the side of the pool so that your feet are at the bottom and toes against the pool's side. Keep your body straight and use your arms to push yourself to and from the pool's side. Alternate slow and fast push-aways.

Explanation

This exercise is pointless unless you tuck your hips and unless your head, your hips, and your seat are always in line with the heels of the feet. If the position is maintained, and if you want to increase the challenge, stand farther from the wall each time you repeat the exercise.

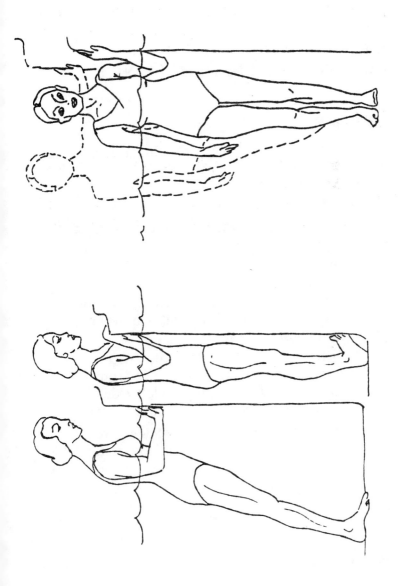

LEG STRAIGHTENER

Starting Position

Stand erect in waist deep or shoulder deep water.

Movements

1. Stand on your right leg. With your right hand, grasp the arch of your left foot and hold it close to you in front of your body.

2. Very slowly stretch and straighten the bent leg in front of you until it is straight as you hold your foot.

3. Still holding the left foot, with leg extended, either keep the leg in front of you or slowly swing it to the left side and hold the position for five or more seconds.

4. Reverse the exercise so that you stretch and extend your right leg while you stand on the left one.

Explanation and Caution

Seldom are people able to keep both legs straight when they first do this exercise. With long (maybe short) practice you should learn to straighten both the supporting leg and the extended working leg. If you have any problem with a hip do not do this exercise.

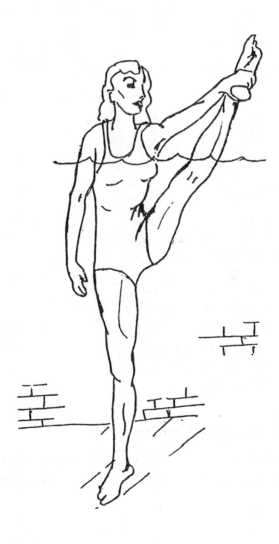

STANDING LEG STRETCHES

Starting Position

Stand erect on both legs in waist deep or shoulder deep water.

Movements

1. Stand on your right leg and bend your left knee so that the knee points to the bottom of the pool. The leg is bent so that the heel of the foot touches the buttock.

2. Hold the ankle in this position a full thirty seconds.

3. Reverse the movements so that you stand on your right leg and bend your left knee. Hold the position as before.

Explanation and Caution

If you have bad knee problems it is suggested you not do this exercise. You must not let your body bend forward or backward. Stand straight at all times. Only the leg moves.

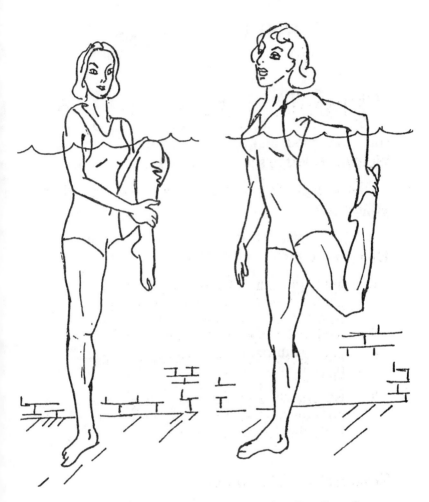

Knee Hugger   Standing Leg Stretches

KNEE HUGGERS

Starting Position

Stand erect with your back against the pool wall. If you have good or average balance, stand erect and without support in shoulder or waist deep water.

Movements

1. Raise you left leg and clasp the calf and ankle areas with both hands -- hug with your arms. Pull your leg hard to your chest while you support yourself on your right leg.

2. Lower the left leg to starting position.

3. Raise your right leg and hug the lower half of the leg with both arms. Hug to the chest; then return to standing position. Repeat the exercise at least three times on each leg.

SHOULDER GIRDLES

Version #1

Starting Position

Stand straight with your whole back against the pool wall. If you are in shallow water, press your feet against the wall and bend your knees away from the wall. You may want to press one or both feet flat up against the wall.

Movements

1. Rotate or roll both shoulders forward and backward.

2. Shrug your shoulders upward and then relax.

3. Shrug or rotate your shoulders downward as smoothly and continuously as you can to the starting position. Repeat these movements at least five times.

Explanation

On the downward movement, press your shoulders to the wall as much as possible. Throughout the rotation be sure that the muscles of the upper spine are not tensed, preventing freedom of movement and a range of motion. The exercise helps mobility of the shoulder girdle and it relieves tension in the neck and shoulder area.

Version #2

Starting Position

Bend your elbows and clasp your hands behind your head as you stand straight.

Movements

1. Using the force from the other hand, pull your arm in the opposite direction and at the same time, resist. Keep your back straight.
2. Reverse arm positions and repeat the exercise several times.

Explanation

This is a resistive exercise to strengthen muscles of your upper back and shoulder girdle. It may be done while you sit at your desk or while you are in the water.

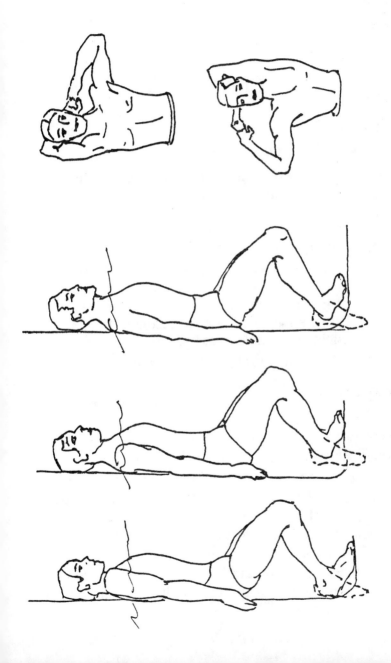

FLATBACK

Starting Position

Stand very erect with your back against the pool wall in waist deep water. Arms are at the sides.

Movements

1. Press your whole back, from your tailbone to the top of your shoulders and neck against the pool wall and hold in your stomach for six to twelve seconds. Inhale deeply and hold your breath.

2. Relax and slowly exhale. Try to breathe out every bit of air.

3. Repeat the movements at least five times.

Explanation

This is very good for the spine, the stomach and the posture. Challenge yourself to inhale deeply, to hold your breath for ten counts as you hold in your stomach, and to exhale even after you think you have pushed out all the air. You may find it easier to bend the knees while you are in this position; it often helps to flatten the back against the wall. Let your lower jaw relax as you open your mouth; breathe through your mouth only.

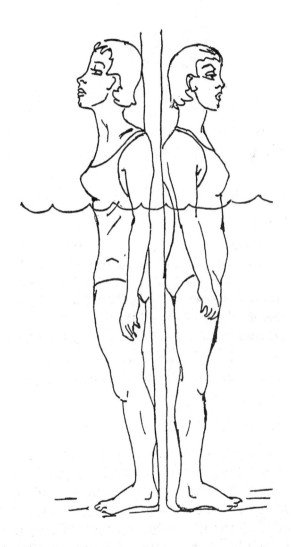

TORSO SWING

Starting Position

Stand straight in waist deep or chest deep water with one side a few inches from the pool wall. Brace yourself with the hand closest to the pool gutter by bending the elbow, or let the arm stay close to the side.

Movements

1. As you straighten the poolside supporting arm, bend your waist away from the poolside so that your body is pulled like a bow. Swing the free, outside arm over your head to further stretch your side.

2. Pull the supporting arm in close to the pool wall and at the same time, swing your waist to the wall. Straighten the free arm out at shoulder height and kick your outside leg so that the toe meets your fingertips.

3. Return to starting position, and repeat this exercise ten times on one side.

4. Reverse your position so that you kick with the former supporting leg and work the other side of your body.

Explanation

This exercise should be done precisely but rapidly.
You can get a lot of benefit from simply bending your
body in and out, to and from the poolside without kicking.

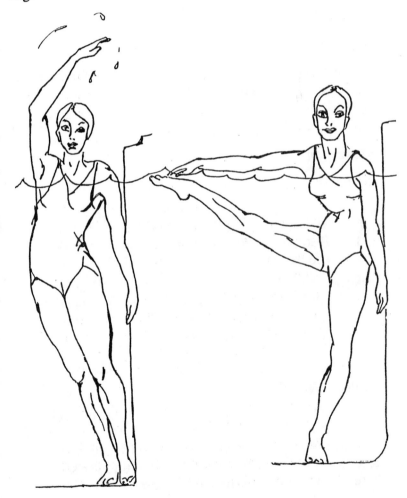

SIDE STRETCHES

Starting Position

In waist deep water, stand with your feet together (or apart with legs kept straight), and left hand on your hip or behind your back.

Movements

1. Bend your torso to the left, try to touch the water's surface with your right fingers.

2. Slowly press three times to the water.

3. Return to standing position; then repeat the exercise three times to the left.

4. Reverse the positions of your arms. Place your left hand over your head and your right hand on your hip. Do the movements the same number of times.

Explanation

Bend the head in the same direction as the body. Be careful not to lean backward or forward. The left arm falls to the right (over the head) and the right arm falls to the left in order to help the body bend far sideways. Stretch until you feel the sides of the torso pull hard.

Variation

Relax one arm. Slide the other hand down from the hip to the thigh as you bend. Stand erect, and repeat the movement with the other hand and arm.

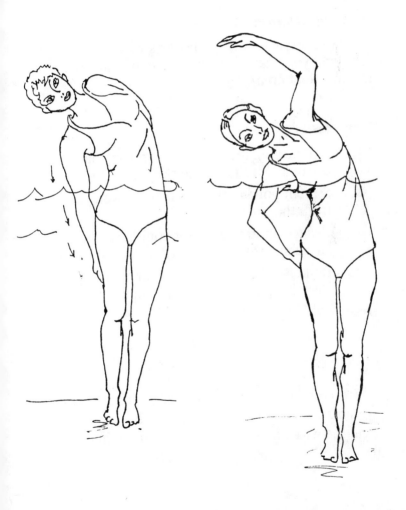

ARM SWINGS

Starting Position

Stand straight with your arms directly above your head and your hands clasped. Keep your legs straight and your feet apart.

Movements

1. Extend your arms above your head, hands clasped. Stretch to the sky.

2. Stretch your arms and bend to your left from the waist.

3. Bring your arms up over your head again, stretching slowly and hard.

4. Bend to the right from your waist, still stretching arms overhead. Repeat a minimum of five times to each side.

Explanation

Remain stretched out the whole time. You must stretch so hard that you feel the pull in the underarm area, the waist, and down the sides at all times.

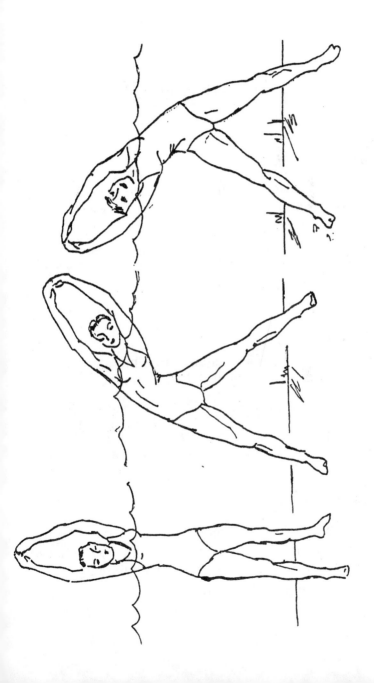

SHOULDER FLEXES

Starting Positions

Partner A spreads his arms as he/she stands erect. Partner B stands behind him and with his right hand he holds A's right wrist (or elbow) and with his left hand he holds A's left wrist (or elbow). Instead of holding partner B's wrist, partner A may hold B's elbows. In which case, A folds her hands behind her head.

Movements

1. Partner B pulls A's arms or elbows; tries to make them meet. B loosens and relaxes his hold and then pulls again. This is done at least three times.

2. Partners change positions and A pulls B's arms or elbows in the same way.

Explanation and Caution

Some people have greater shoulder flexibility than others; how far back the arms will go varies greatly. Always keep in mind that you should very gently and slowly stretch your partner. NEVER bounce, jerk or force his/her arms. Partner A should remain erect all the time his arms are being stretched behind him; he should not slump forward. *NEVER DO THIS EXERCISE IF YOU HAVE ANY SHOULDER PROBLEMS.*

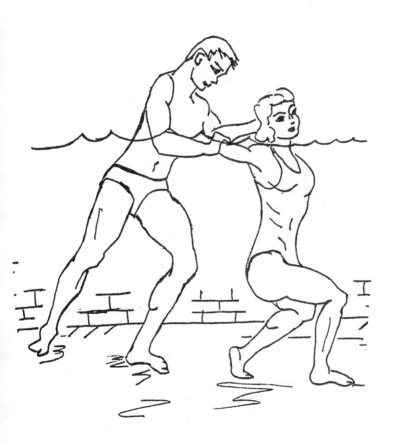

PATTIE-CAKE

Starting Position

Partners stand facing each other with the palms of both hands pressing against the palms of the partner.

Movements

1. Each partner pushes forward, and tries to move the other from his/her position.
2. Both partners relax and then repeat the above movement at least three times.

Explanation

Doing this exercise with weights on the wrists will help strengthen the shoulder muscles to enable you to do other exercises or heavy swimming strokes.

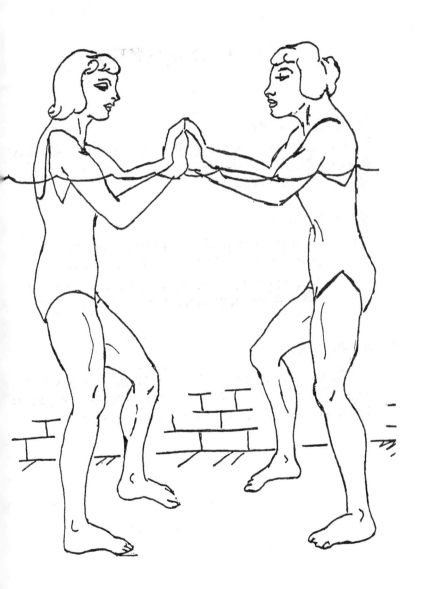

PULLS AND PUSHES

Starting Positions

Partners stand erect, facing each other. They clasp right wrists and one partner braces the outside of his left foot against the inside of his partner's right foot.

Movements

1. Each partner tries to pull the other one off balance to his/her side.
2. Reverse arm and leg positions and repeat the exercise.

Consult Illustration on following page.

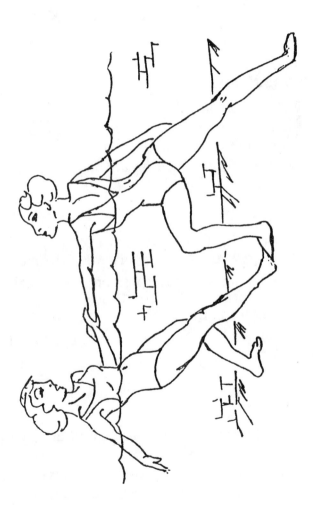

ELBOW CIRCLES

Starting Position

Stand in shoulder deep water, or squat so your shoulders are underwater. Keep your back straight. Extend arms straight out from each shoulder. Now bend your elbows so that your fingertips are on your shoulders.

Movements

1. Keeping the above shoulder position, rotate your elbows forward five times.

2. Keeping the above position, reverse the direction of your elbows' rotation backward, five times.

3. Repeat this set of movements five to ten times.

Explanation

Even if you are in good shape, your arms should be tired when you finish this exercise. It may be done anywhere, but it's most effective when it is done underwater; you get the factor of water resistance.

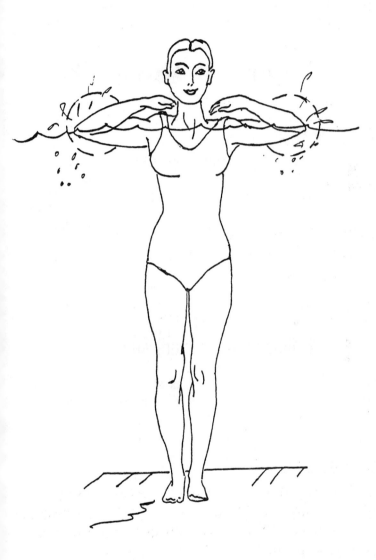

ARM RAISERS AND CIRCLES

Starting Position

Stand erect in shoulder deep water. Be sure that shoulders are under water. If the water is only waist deep, squat so that your shoulders are covered. Bend your legs, but keep your back straight. Begin by having the arms straight down at each side and close to your body.

Movements

1. Make small circles from the fingertips to the shoulders with both arms straight (throughout). As you make the small circles, raise both arms slowly until you have circled them to the surface of the water.

2. Make very large circles from the surface of the water to below the hips or where the arms were in starting position. Do this three times, and keep the arms under the water.

3. Repeat first movement, only reverse the direction of the small as well as the large circles.

Explanation

The exercise may be done simply by extending the straight arms in opposite directions, and it may be done underwater or by breaking the surface of the water when making the large circles.

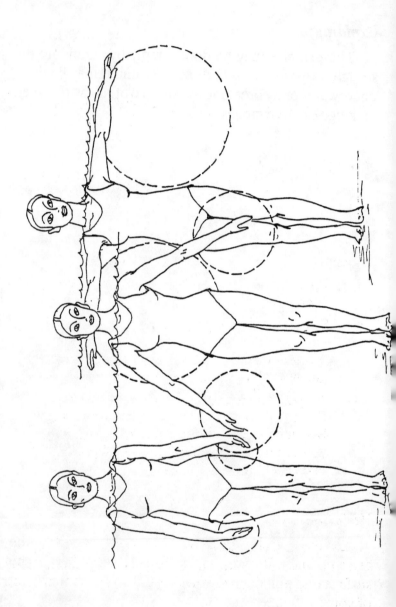

RHYTHMIC ARM CROSSES

Starting Position

Stand erect in waist or shoulder deep water. Spread straight legs comfortably apart.

Movements

1. Raise both arms straight up above your head.

2. Swing the arms straight down to the sides and across in front of you in the water. Swing your arms downward, bend your knees so that you establish a rhythm.

3. As you again straighten your legs swing the arms outward again and upward. Repeat the exercise at least ten times as you establish a definite rhythm by bending and straightening you legs.

Variation

Do the exercise the same way except for raising the arms up and out of the water. Simply raise them to the surface and pull them downward and cross them in front of you.

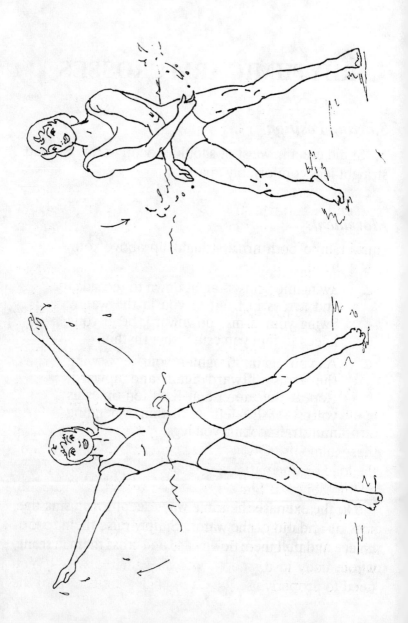

CONDITIONING AND STRETCHING

Start at your head and work down, or start at your feet and work up to stretch all parts of your body. Hold all stretch positions a minimum of ten seconds and a maximum of one minute. *Never* bounce.

Your heartbeat should be lower than your target level. After this section of your program, your pulse rate should be an average of 120 or lower. These exercises may be isometric or isotonic: use kickboards; drill arms and legs using various swimming strokes; do much reaching, pulling, pressing.

As time goes by, a little loss of coordination leads to an increased and greater loss. Deep centers of control atrophy and we adjust by sitting more and compounding these ailments. Often people compensate by lightening the load on one part of the body and increasing the load on another part. Simple, wrong action can reach up into the neck, and nerves knot up. Of course, rest, massage, special attentions may make you temporarily comfortable. What you really need is to learn how to use the whole body in a smooth and coordinated way. You need to properly use the offendingly painful part of the body and make it perform or function correctly so that it will not create compound complications. Begin by knowing something basic about two main movements in the body: the horizontal and the vertical.

The horizontal movements go crosswise, i.e., from the hip joint to the hip joint, from rib to rib and from shoulder to shoulder. The muscles take a pattern and form of the figure 8. For example, imagine a dot in the center of the pelvis (the last vertebra of the spine in the back) and the pubic bone in front. These two points are the center from which movement flows in a figure 8. There are four main movement centers of control -- horizontally.

1. The head center controls the face and the head. It is the most sensitive and delicate of all because it involves the important and fine nerves as well as the bone and muscle structures of the head.

2. The neck center controls the neck and the connections of the head and body. It is next in delicate sensitivity.

3. The arms and diaphragm center controls the rib area, the shoulders, arms and hands. This, with the upper back and chest muscles, is the second strongest part of the body.

4. The pelvic-led center controls the lower regions, the hips, legs, and feet. This is the strongest part of the bone and muscle structure of the body.

The vertical movement of the body is dominated by the spinal column that passes through each vertebra and each sequence. When it functions properly it connects the four centers in an up and down action. It keeps the muscles of the torso flexible.

When both horizontal and vertical movement centers function healthily, your body is in balance and you have a feeling of vitality and well-being. Most people, however, move only a small part of their original capacity for movement; so they need deep and conscious exercises as well as deep breathing to preserve or to restore their flexibility and stretching capacities.

For our purposes, the main properties of muscles include extensibility, elasticity, contractility, and amplitude.

Extensibility refers to the stretchable nature of muscles' fiber as distinct from ligaments and tendons that are not usually extensible in average movements. Muscle fiber can be stretched one-third to one-half beyond its normal resting length. We need to use muscles to keep them in this condition; however, one needs to be very cautious, for if we create sudden, strong, force in order to stretch our muscles farther, we are likely to rupture them. Abnormal force can rupture the junction of the muscle fibers into the tendon of insertion. Capillaries also may rupture and we get something like a bruise, a black and blue spot. Even though a repaired muscle may be very strong, it loses some of its original flexibility if it is thus injured. It never can be as good as it was originally.

Recoil from a stretch is known as elasticity. Like a rubber band, a normal muscle snaps back after it is stretched, yet this recoil never is a hundred percent. Contractility compensates for the less than one hundred percent elastic recoil, and it produces movement or control position of the body. Contractility is possible in muscles up to one-third to one-half of the resting length of the muscle fibers. Most physical educators classify a muscle according to the movement produced by its concentric contraction.

People often ask, "How much should I stretch?" The answer depends upon understanding the amplitude of a muscle or the range through which it can operate from its most completely stretched position or extended position, through elastic recoil and full concentric contraction. Amplitude of a muscle is normally seventy to one hundred percent of its fibrous portion's (not its tendinous portion's) resting length.

Normally, muscles are adequate in amplitude and long enough to let them move bones through the normal range of joint movements. The less a person uses this full range of muscle movement, muscle amplitude decreases. Finally, lack of use can cause muscles to be impotent. They can not stretch out fully or contract adequately. If a person suddenly or forcefully attempts to make a muscle operate its original range of movement, that muscle may rupture. Obviously, when a person who has not exercised -- moves muscles through their range -- for a long time, tries to perform movements that strain an unused muscle, that muscle may have its fibers ruptured. If this is not bad enough, there's more, the muscle never again will regain its normal movement.

Be careful. Remember that when a muscle fiber is stretched, it normally responds by contracting. This is called stretch reflex.

How can one improve his muscles' performance? Many authorities believe the way to increase strength is by overloading muscles by use of weights, by changes of body position, by isometrics, and by tempo. Water exercises gently overload the muscles through the weight and the resistance of the water, by using exercises to change body positions, by isometrics, and by tempo.

Aquacises help you attain both strength and muscular power. You develop strength through raising your body weight from a squatting to an erect position or by raising your leg with a leg lift. You develop power, however, when you suddenly apply enough momentum to raise your body from the bottom of the pool into a leap or a jump. The higher you jump, the greater the power. In other words, you develop elasticity, contractility, amplitude and strength of muscles by practicing conditioning and stretching water exercises.

You develop power when you practice water aerobic exercises. Only after you have warmed up your muscles is it safe to do the exercises in this section. These exercises should be performed before you move on to do the aerobics.

FRUSTRATED BALL

Starting Position

Firmly grasp the pool gutter with both hands. Plant your feet as close to your hands as possible with, the feet positioned outside the hands and the knees fully bent into a squatting position. Your back is rounded and your knees are pointed in opposite directions.

Movement

Maintain this starting position throughout the exercise. Pull with your hands and arms so that you make your forehead press against the pool gutter. You should look like a frustrated ball, your head, hands, and your feet should be close to the gutter and pressed against the poolside. Your forehead is between your hands, and your hands are between your feet. Hold this position for the count of ten -- slow counts. Relax, but maintain the position of the feet, hands, and knees. Repeat the pull as you again touch your forehead to the poolside. Repeat this exercise at least five times.

Explanation

Stretch firmly, steadily, and slowly. Never jerk. This exercise helps firm the inside of the legs and groin areas, For variety you may spread your straight legs apart.

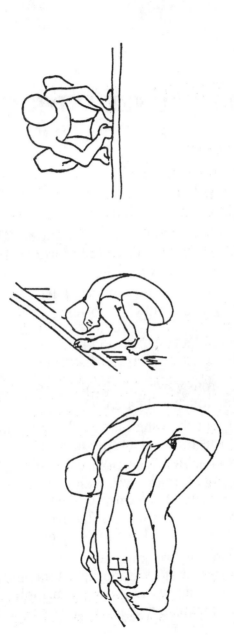

BENT KNEE AND KICK COMBINATION

Starting Position

Stand straight, your side facing the pool and your inside (pool side) hand holding the gutter. The leg near the pool remains straight and supporting. The working leg, away from the poolside, is bent so that the toe touches the knee of the supporting leg. Of course, the working leg is bent outward, forming a triangle.

Movements

1. Vigorously swing the bent knee so that the knee touches the pool wall.

2. Vigorously swing the bent knee so that it returns to starting position.

3. Without dropping the level of the knee, kick and then straighten the leg hard, upward and outward. The toe of the working leg moves swiftly from touching the supporting knee to being elevated.

4. Bend the working leg so that the toe returns to starting position touching the supporting knee. Without dropping the toe from the level of the supporting knee,

repeat the exercise ten times; then reverse
leg positions so that the supporting leg
becomes the working leg. When you
reverse the exercise, you must turn so that
you face the opposite direction. For
example, you may begin the exercise by
facing the shallow end of the pool;then
you turn to face the deep end of the pool.

Variation

The exercise may be simplified by simply keeping
the working leg bent and swinging it in and out from the
pool wall. Likewise, the straightened leg may be lifted
and then swung in and out, from and to the wall. You
could do five bent swings and five straight leg swings for
a change.

Explanation

Although you may tire, do not drop the level of the
working toe or knee at any time during the exercise of
one leg. Count to yourself rhythmically.

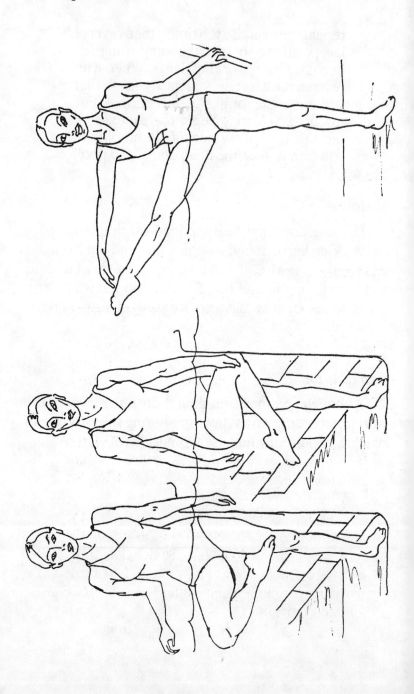

HIP TWIST LIFT

Starting Position

Stand straight with your side to the pool wall and one hand holding the gutter for balance.

Movements

1. The supporting and the working leg must both be kept straight. Swing the working leg (leg away from the wall) straight up from the side, first with the leg twisted so that the instep and the toe are up and the inside of the leg and the hip are turned outward.

2. Swing the leg down to starting position.

3. Keeping both legs straight, swing the working leg high with the heel of the foot turned upward and the inside of the leg turned down and inward.

4. Swing the leg ten times alternating the inward and the outward positions of the leg and foot with each swing.

5. Reverse so that the working leg is the supporting leg and repeat the exercise ten times.

Explanation

As you become increasingly proficient you will swing the leg higher; however, you should sacrifice the height of the leg swing to the proper position of the leg and hips. This exercise not only strengthens the legs and helps posture, it also exercises and limbers the hips. If you have a hip replacement or problems with the hips, avoid executing this exercise.

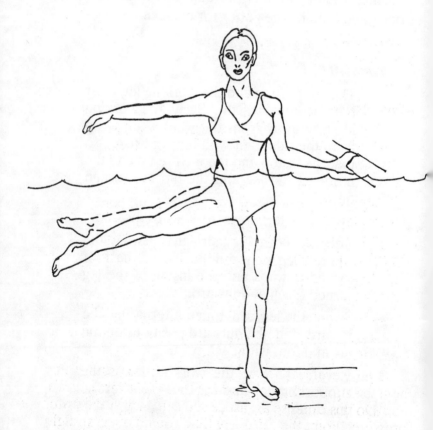

MIXED LEG LIFTS

Starting Position

Stand right beside the pool wall, one side near the wall with one hand on the ledge of the gutter for support. Stand erect and look straight ahead during the exercise. Your feet and your legs are together.

Movements

1. Lift your very straight leg (the leg away from the wall) and lower it. Pull all your muscles and point your toe hard.

2. Continue to use the same working leg, away from the wall. Bend the knee hard and at the same time raise the knee, and point your toe hard as it leaves the bottom of the pool.

3. Reverse your position so that you work the leg that has been supporting you.

Explanation

You will alternate lifting a straight leg and lifting bent leg, up and down: lift straight, down, lift bent, down, etc. Do this exercise as fast as you can against the water pressure. Point the toe every time you lift a leg, straight or bent.

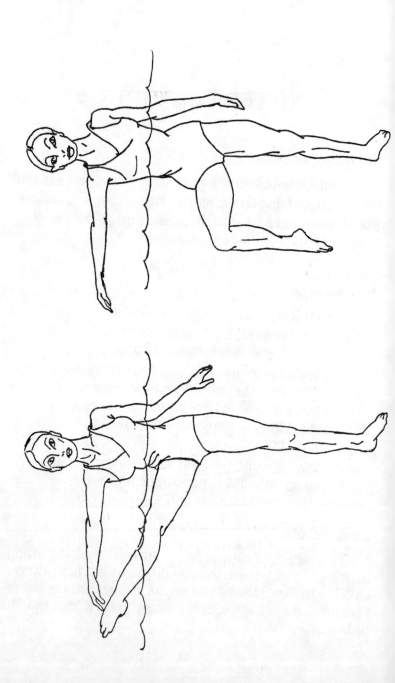

HIP TWISTER

Starting Position

Stand straight with your back against the pool wall and your arms outstretched along the gutter. You should be in waist deep to shoulder deep water.

Movements

1. Pull up your knees into a squatting position. Continue to keep your back against the side of the pool.

2. Keeping your bent legs together, twist from the waist to your right so that your hips turn as far as possible.

3. Return to starting position, legs together and bent.

4. Keeping your body straight and against the side of the pool, legs together and bent, twist from the waist to your left so that your hips turn as far as possible.

5. Return to starting position.

6. Repeat five times to one side and five times to the other side.

Explanation

Again, it is important that each movement be precisely executed in spite of doing this exercise swiftly. Do not sacrifice form for speed.

Variation

Add zest and aerobics to this exercise by doing it away from the wall. Jump on both feet each time you twist and alternate twisting from one side to the other. Jump -- twist right -- jump -- twist left -- etc.

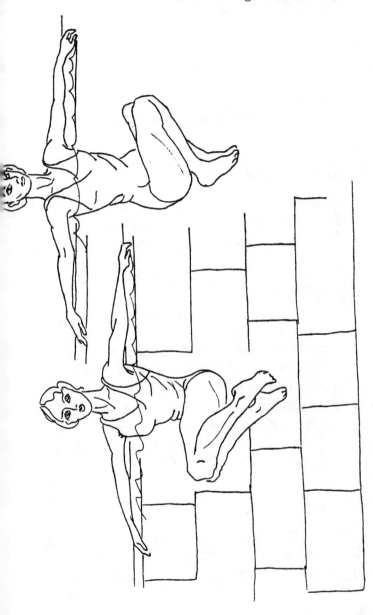

SWINGAROO

Starting Position

Stand straight, legs and feet together, in chest deep water. The exercise may be done either bracing against the pool wall or standing away from the wall.

Movements

1. The movements should originate at the waist. Continue to stand in the same place and swing the top of your torso, head and shoulders, to the right, and the bottom of your torso, hips and legs, to the left.

2. Reverse the movements so that you swing the top of your torso, head and shoulders, to the left, and the bottom of your torso, hips and legs, to the right.

Explanation

Your arms may extend above the water along the gutter. Do this exercise very fast for a full minute. After you understand it and can do it slowly, increase your speed.

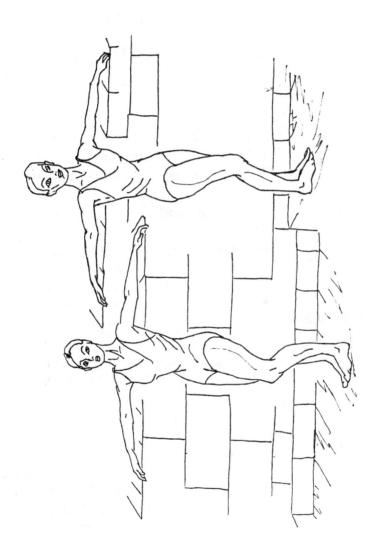

DOUBLE LEG CIRCLES

Starting Position

You may start this exercise from either of two positions. You may start by lying flat on your back with your hands close to your ears and holding onto the gutter or you may stand straight with your legs, body, and shoulders against the pool wall and your arms extending in opposite directions along the gutter. Whichever position you use to begin your exercise you should also be in when you finish it.

Movements

1. From either the surface of the water or from the bottom of the pool, raise your legs together without bending the knees.

2. Swing the legs vigorously; pivot them from your hips and waist so that they make a complete circle, moving from the surface or out of the water, to the side, to the bottom of the pool, up and over the water, back to the water's surface. Or move the legs in a circle from the bottom of the pool, to your right; swing them straight up and over the water's surface, then down the left side to the bottom again. Move

the legs so that you complete at least five full circles.

3. Circle the legs in the reverse direction for a minimum of five times. If you begin with the clockwise circles, then you move them in the counter-clockwise circles.

Explanation

Each circle must be carefully and completely made so that your toes touch the pool bottom and so that they also rise perpendicular over the water's surface.

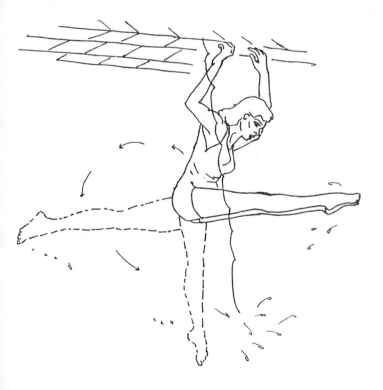

CYCLING

Starting Position

Lie on your back with your arms outstretched or bent and holding onto the gutter with your arms held alongside your ears -- whichever is comfortable.

Movements

1. Start to cycle slowly and then increase and/or alter your speed for thirty seconds.

2. Cycle backward. Instead of pushing the foot downward, pull the leg upward, as if to brake on an old-fashioned bicycle without hand brakes.

3. Turn on the right side and continue to cycle (regular) for at least thirty seconds. Increase your speed.

4. Turn on your left side and continue to cycle (regular) for at least thirty seconds.

5. Return to the back position and cycle a few seconds.

Explanation

Vigorous cycling may substitute for aerobic exercise.

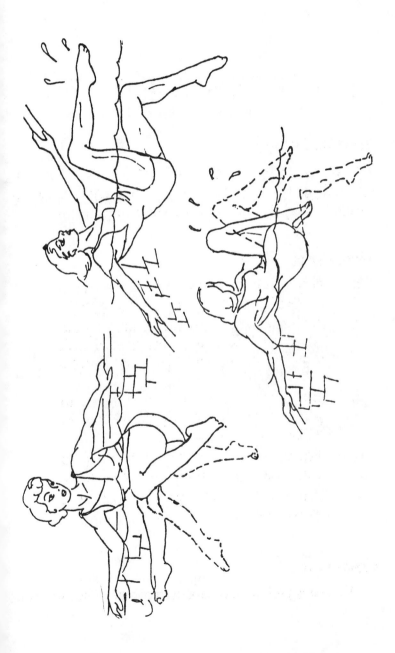

BARRE: BACK LEG EXERCISES

Warning

People who have back or hip problems should not attempt these exercises. They are adapted from ballet barre exercises.

Starting Position

Stand erect with one side to the pool wall. Steady yourself by holding one hand on the pool gutter or side. Keep your back and both legs straight throughout this exercise. Keep your hips at right angles to the pool (or parallel if back or front is to the pool) and keep your feet and your hips turned out. Do not roll onto the inside of the foot.

Movements

1. As you stand on your right leg, swing your left leg high so that the heel of your foot touches the gutter.

2. Keeping your hips at right angles to the gutter and continuing to stand parallel to the wall with the supporting foot turned

out, swing your leg to the rear so that part of the foot is supported by the gutter.

3.   Return to starting position.

4.   Swing the leg from top high front position to back high position. Alternate front and back positions five times front, and five times back. Reverse legs. Attempt to hold the high leg positions for a couple of seconds; do not simply drop leg.

Explanation

While the leg is in high front position, be sure to keep your body erect; do not tilt backward. While the leg swings to the back position, be sure to keep your shoulders up and your body perpendicular to the poolside; do *not* bend forward. Be very aware of form on this exercise. If the leg does not go high, do not force height by bending the body. Keep the supporting leg straight and the feet and hips always turned out. Be sure that the working leg (the one that rises forward and backward) is away from the wall. Note how the arm swings forward for balancing when the leg is swung back. When the leg is swung forward, the arm should be held about shoulder height and directly out to the side.

This may be difficult for beginners; so do not expect to get the leg high or to do this exercise well the first few times. Again, do not sacrifice form. Be patient and practice will enable you to lift that leg high after awhile.

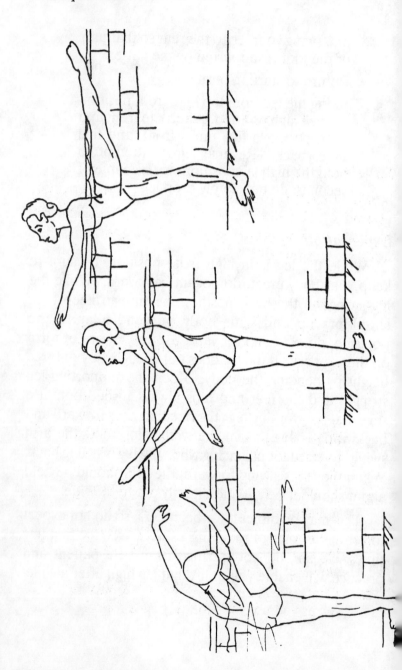

LEG STRETCHES

Starting Position

Stand erect in chest deep water with one side to the pool wall and one hand resting on the pool gutter for support. As you become increasingly expert, you may not need this support.

Movements

1. Keep the supporting leg straight. Bend the working leg and grasp the arch of the working foot.

2. Still holding the arch of the foot, straighten the working leg in front of you and at the same time swing the leg widely to the side. Fully straighten the working leg and aim to extend it up to your ear. If you can not do this, then extend it as far as you can.

3. As you fully straighten the working leg, pull and hold it for a slow count of 1-2-3.

4. Do not drop, but try to hold the extended leg and let it go down slowly. Lower it as slowly as possible.

5. Change legs and exercise the supporting leg as you use the other leg for support.

Explanation

At first you likely will not be able to extend your leg higher than your waist, but with practice you will go higher. Often one leg is more flexible than the other. I suggest working first with the "bad" leg and doing at least one extra exercise with that leg.

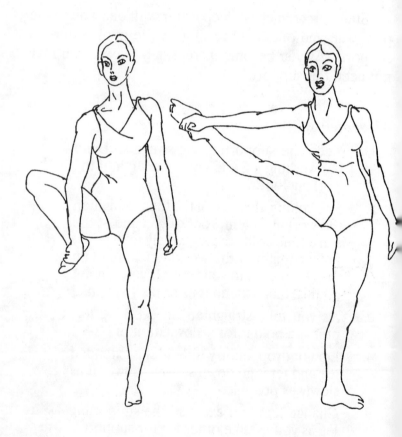

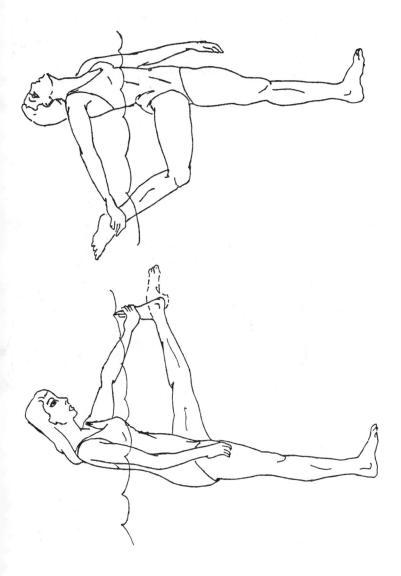

BACK/LEG STRETCH

Warning

Do not do this exercise if you have lower back problems.

Starting Position

Stand erect with one side to the pool wall and one hand resting on the pool gutter for support. As you become expert, you may not need this support.

Movements

1. Grasp the ankle of the working leg and hold it behind you. The working leg is bent.

2. Still holding the ankle, stretch the working leg directly to the rear. Try to straighten the leg as you hold it. Try to pull the toes up to the back of your head. Relax. Do the exercise three times minimum.

3. Change legs and repeat the exercise.

Variation

A variation of this exercise is to hold the working knee; for example, hold the right knee firmly to one side with the right hand. Twist your waist so that your toe that was pointed downward, points directly behind you. As you continue to clasp your knee, your leg and foot extend upward and outward as your back arches. In both versions, the emphasis is upon working for a back arch.

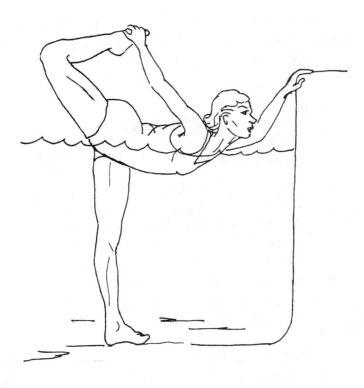

CRISS/CROSSES

Starting Position

Lie flat on your back on top of the water and hold the pool gutter with both hands, arms extended behind you. Your legs are together and straight in front of you.

Movements

1. Spread your legs in splits fashion, in opposite directions. Keep your legs straight and your toes pointed.

2. Pull your straight legs together to starting position.

3. Swing your right leg over your left leg and spread them, scissorlike, as far apart as possible.

4. Return to starting position.

5. Swing your left leg over your right leg and spread them as far apart as possible.

6. Return to starting position.

7. Repeat the series of movements for at least one minute.

Explanation

This exercise may be broken down so that you simply do the leg crosses, one side and then the other side quickly, or you may simply want to alternately spread the legs in splits and bring them together repeatedly.

The legs must be kept straight at all times and the toes must be pointed. The faster the exercise is done and the more resistance of the water you feel, the more benefit you will receive.

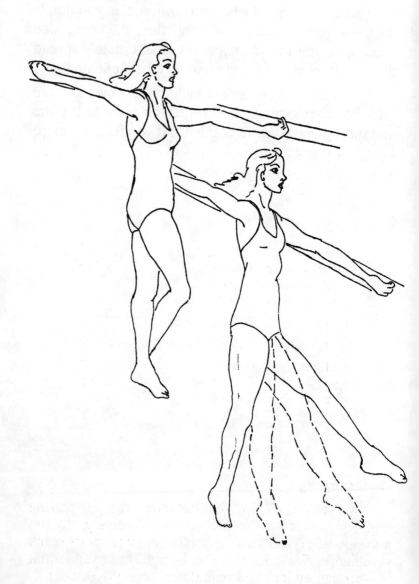

POOL WALL WALK

Starting Position

Stand erect facing the side of the pool. Place both hands on the gutter or top of pool. Step backward so that you are arms' length from the side.

Movements

1. Keep the legs straight throughout the execution of this exercise. Start walking -- take small steps up the side of the pool -- while you continue to hold to the gutter.

2. Keeping the legs straight, take small steps and walk down to the bottom of the pool.

3. Repeat the up and down walking at least seven times. Be sure to walk the feet up to meet the hands at the top of the water each time. Keep the feet flat against the wall.

Variation

You may combine this exercise with Hamstring Squatting Exercise by pulling your bent legs to the poolside after you have walked your feet up to reach your hands. Walk down the wall -- bend knees and squat in -- straighten legs and walk down the wall. Repeat.

HAMSTRING SQUATTING STRETCHES

Starting Position

Face the poolside and hold the pool gutter with both hands. Place your feet flat against the poolside, close to your hands, and assume a frog-like squat against the side.

Movements

1. Slowly straighten your bent knees so that your legs are straight and your feet are flat, close to your hands, at the top of the pool wall. Hold the position for ten long counts.

2. Relax and resume the bent knee, squat position.

3. Again slowly straighten your knees so that the legs are straight. Keeping the legs straight and the feet flat as possible, walk down the wall to the bottom of the pool.

4. Walk up the pool's side so that your feet again are close to your hands.

5. Bend and relax your legs; then straighten them, stretch, then walk up and down the pool wall, stiff-legged, at least three times.

Explanation

As in the case of all stretching exercises, this stretch must be done slowly but steadily. Unless the knees are fully straightened and unless the feet are close to the hands, the exercise is pointless. The bending and straightening, and the walking up and down the pool wall may be alternated in any way that pleases you, e.g., five stretches and bends and then five Pool Wall Walks, or five sets of walking, stretching and bending. Keep the feet flat against the wall at all times.

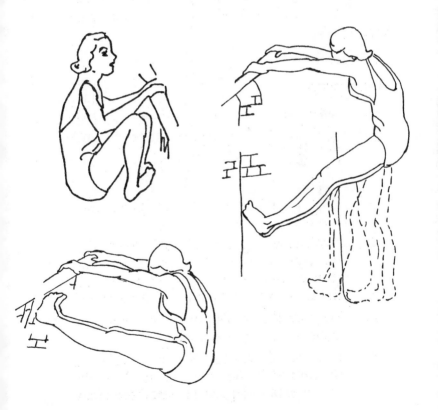

STANDING LEG CROSSES

Starting Position

Stand straight, legs together and arms out along the pool gutter. You are facing the water, your back against the side of the pool.

Movements

1. Keeping the supporting leg straight, lift your left leg as high as possible. Keep the leg straight and stretched in front of you.

2. Swing your left leg to the left so that the leg is parallel to your outstretched left arm.

3. Without lowering the height of the working leg, swing it forward and then swing it across your body so that your left foot touches the poolside at your right.

4. Swing the left leg so that it is straight, but directly in front of you at the height you have (hopefully) maintained; then lower the leg.

5. Repeat the whole exercise by reversing legs. The left leg will support you and the right leg will swing, or be the working leg. Repeat the exercise so that you do a minimum of five leg crosses with each leg.

Explanation

Even though this may be a good out of the water exercise, it is a better in the water exercise because you get the extra benefit from the resistance of the water against the moving leg. Try to do this swiftly. Buoyancy will help you to keep your working leg elevated.

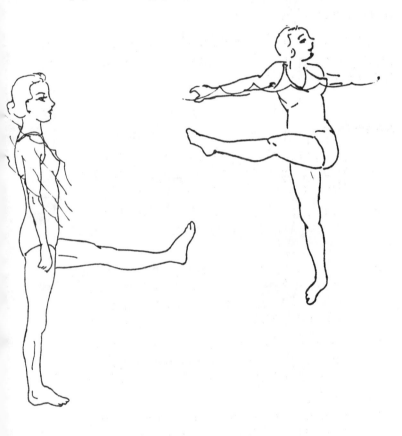

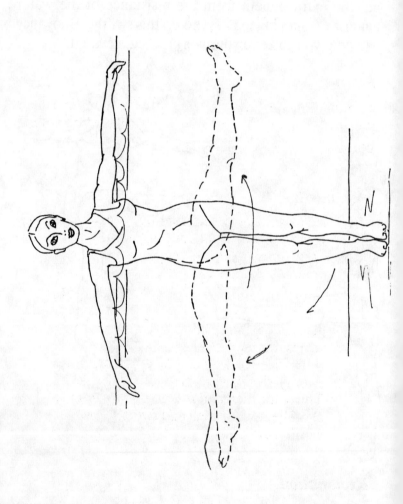

DECK PUSH-UPS

Starting Position

Stand in chest deep water and face the pool's deck. Place your hands flat on top of the deck, close to your body.

Movements

1. Relax your body and use your arms to lift your entire, straight body out of the water. Your arms should straighten as your body emerges, usually to the hips.

2. Your straightened arms should support the rest of your body for several counts, at least to ten. The number of push-ups varies: for men, seventy-five are excellent; thirty-five for women. Fifty for men and twenty-five for women are very good. Thirty for men and fifteen for women are average, ten for men and five or fewer for women are poor.

Explanation

If the pool deck is high and if it has a moderately high gutter, you may begin this exercise by using the gutter for a pushing base; however, you should gradually learn to use the deck. You lose the benefits of this shoulder,arm and chest building exercise if you do it in shallow water and if you bounce hard with your feet from the bottom; your shoulders and arms should carry and hold your weight; so do this in chest deep water. Hold each push-up for at least three counts and be certain the arms are straight and your body is suspended between your arms. People with shoulder problems should not do it.

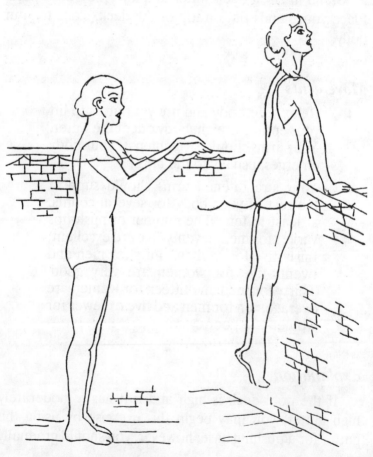

DECK SIT-UPS

Starting Position

Water depth is not important for this exercise. Hold onto the deck or pool gutter with both hands and place your forelegs together over the top of the deck. Your knees bend so that the forelegs lie on top of the deck and your thighs are perpendicular to the deck as you lie on your back, head back on top of the water.

Movements

1. (Beginners) Grasp the poolside or the gutter firmly and pull your body upward so that your chest touches your thighs.

2. Relax and return to prone position from the hips to the head.

3. Repeat by again and again pulling your chest to your thighs and then relaxing. Put the strain on your stomach rather than on your arm muscles. The usual ten repetitions of the cycle is recommended for everyone.

Explanation

More advanced people may fold their hands behind their heads, elbows extended in opposite directions, and do the entire lift with the stomach muscles. Do this exercise completely, so that your entire back is out of the water on each exercise. This is not recommended for pregnant women or for those who have recently had abdominal surgery. It is recommended for those who have adhesions or flabby abdominal muscles.

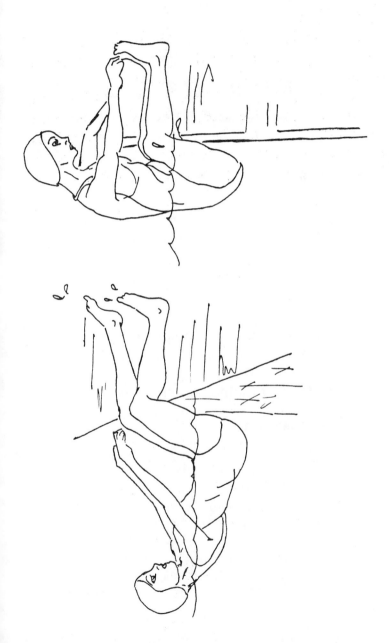

HAMSTRING STANDING STRETCHES

Starting Position

Stand straight, your arms at your sides, about six to eight inches from the pool wall. Face the pool wall as you do the exercise. Continue to gaze straight ahead; do not look downward or upward.

Movements

1. Pull your hands upward, close into your body, palms out.

2. Keeping the back straight and the heels of the feet on the bottom, let your body fall against the poolside, The palms of your hands take the impact.

3. Push yourself forcefully from the pool wall; now you can continue to grasp the poolside or gutter.

4. Keeping your heels down, your legs and your back straight, push yourself back and forth, to and from the poolside, rapidly and hard. Feel the water's resistance and the stretch up the back of your legs. Continue for a minimum of thirty seconds.

Variation

Pull your whole body up as close as possible to the pool wall. Position your feet so that your heels are on the bottom and your arches and toes are up against the pool wall. Quickly push your straight body in and out from the wall, but keep your feet in their original positions.

Explanation

The point of the exercise is lost if your back end protrudes, even slightly. Your back must be kept aligned, and there must be a straight line from the heels of your feet to the nap of your neck. Likewise, the heels of the feet must be down, feet flat at all times. After you have done one or two stretches, step a few feet farther from the wall to increase the challenge and the stretch. You should feel the hamstrings pull if you do this properly.

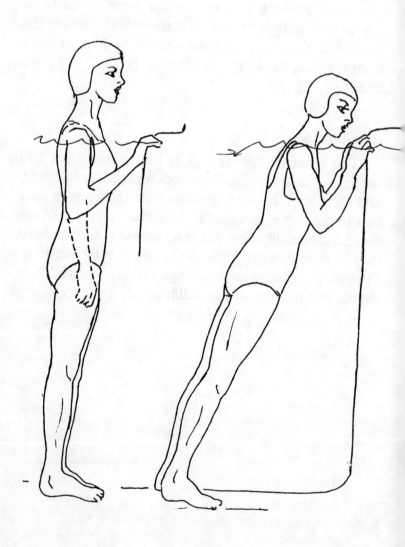

THREE-WAY STRETCH

Starting Position

Stand straight facing the side of the pool with both hands lightly holding the gutter for balance.

Movements

1. Stand on the left leg and keep it straight throughout the execution of this exercise. Hump your back and bend the right knee and try to touch your knee to your nose.

2. Quickly thrust the right leg directly behind you into a straightened position. As you push the leg backward, pull your head up and arch your back.

3. Without lowering the right leg (at any time), bend the knee again and pull the knee to one side as if you were trying to touch your knee to your ear. The inside of bent, right leg should be parallel to the pool bottom.

4. Return to starting position, both feet on the bottom.

5. Reverse the whole set of movements so that you are moving the left leg and you are using the right leg in the supporting

capacity. Alternating legs, do this set of movements five times on each leg.

Variation

1. As you begin movement number three, do not bring the knee to the ear, but try to touch the right toe to the wall at your left side as you keep the knee elevated. If you are exercising the left leg, you will try to touch the wall to your right.

2. Very quickly tuck your knee to your nose and then straighten the leg without touching the knee to the ear or the toe to the opposite wall. Simply duck and straighten the leg rapidly.

3. All three of these versions should be done in waist to chest deep water in order to get the benefit of water resistance.

Explanation

Proper position is important. Make an extra effort to keep the knee elevated.

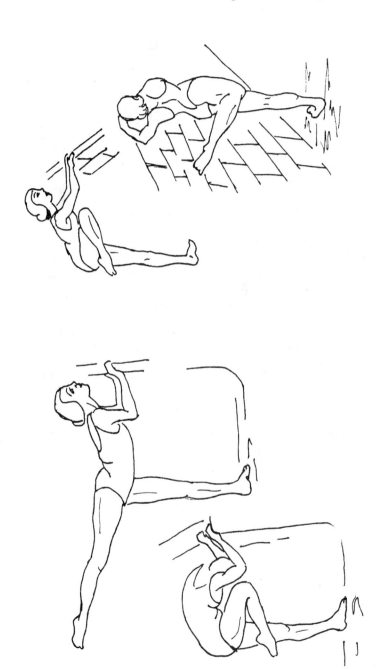

BACK BEND

Starting Position

Stand straight, your back to the poolside.

Movements

1. Lift your hands up and over your head, and at the same time bend the back -- backward.

2. Clasp the gutter and push your tummy upward. Arch your neck and back deeply.

3. Relax and repeat the movement four or five times.

Warning

If you have an injured or problem back or neck do not do this exercise.

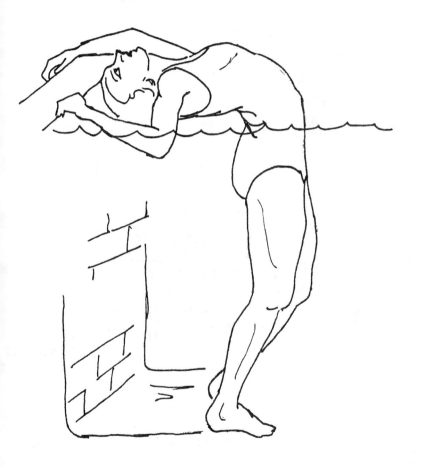

SOLE STRETCHES

Starting Position

Stand in chest deep or waist deep water beside the pool wall. Brace yourself by spreading your arms outward along the deck or gutter. Lie flat on your back on top of the water.

Movements

1. Keep your legs as straight as possible and place the soles of your feet together.

2. Keeping the soles of your feet together at all times, bend your knees upward and outward.

3. Still keeping the soles of your feet together, straighten your legs as much as possible. Repeat these movements at least five times.

Explanation

As you become practiced in this exercise, first do it slowly and then do the movements as fast as you can. Start with several slow cycles; do several very fast cycles, and then do several slow ones again. This helps tighten and firm the inner thighs.

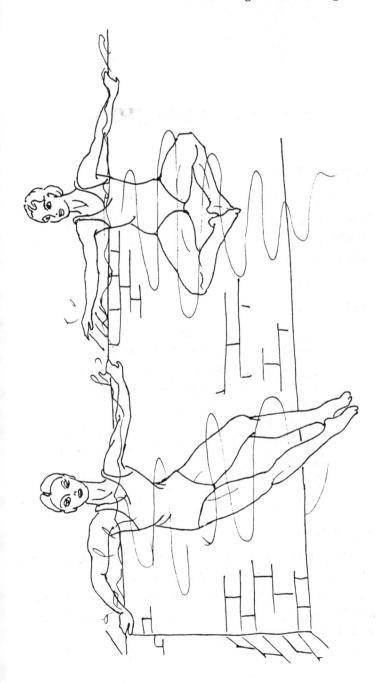

LEG LIFTS

Starting Position

Lie prone -- on your back -- with your legs together and your hands holding the pool gutter beside your ears, elbows bent.

Movements

1. Keeping your back flat, pull your knees up to your chest until your thighs are perpendicular to the surface of the water. Keep the legs together.

2. Lift both legs together and extend them upward so that they are as close to perpendicular to the water's surface as you can manage.

3. Spread your lifted legs to form a wide V, then cross the legs at least three times.

4. Pull the legs together in the upward, extended position.

5. Bend the knees and return to starting position.

Explanation

Use your imagination to create variations of this exercise. For example, you may simply raise the legs to extend them upwards and count first to five and then to ten as your strength develops. You may lift one leg and count and then lift the other leg and count. As your skill increases, you may want to pull the knees up to your chest and then swing your toes back towards the pool wall over your head. The longer you hold you legs in the number two position, and the more slowly you do the exercise, the more you will develop your stomach muscles. Bending the knees in all leg lifts helps to eliminate problems for people who have weak or painful backs. As your stomach muscles strengthen, you will be able to straighten your legs as you lift them without suffering ill effects. This is because you have developed stomach muscles that take the load from the lower back muscles. Try flutterkicking in the air with your raised, straight legs.

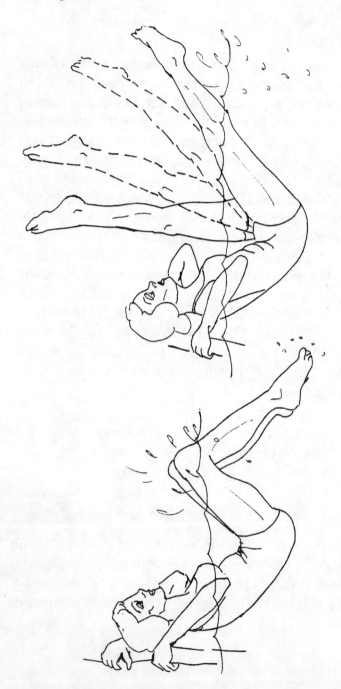

WALK-THROUGH

Starting Position

Stand in waist deep water. The kickboard lies flat on top of the water in front of you. Hold it by a hand on each end.

Movements

1. Bend forward as you firmly grip the board and press it under the water. Do not let go of the board as you first walk one foot and then the other foot through the space between the kickboard and your shoulders.

2. Finally, hold the board securely and jump (both feet at the same time) back and forth over the kickboard at least five times.

Explanation

You may have to learn to do this one, or maybe you will need to lose some rolls from your middle before you do the fast jump through. It helps your balance and it helps a stiff back as well as reduce the sides and stomach rolls.

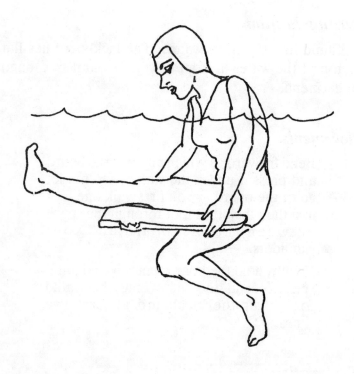

KICKBOARD TOE-TOUCH

Starting Position

Lie on your back as if you were floating and hold the kickboard across your chest and under your arms. Water depth does not matter in this exercise.

Movements

1. Bend from your waist as you pull your arms over the top of the kickboard so that you touch your fingertips to your toes. You move into a sitting position.

2. Return to starting position, lying on your back.

3. Sit up and again touch your toes. Swiftly alternate toe-touching and lying flat on your back for thirty or more times, at least one minute.

Variations

Lie flat on your back and hold the kickboard across your chest. Start by having your legs together; then do these movements:

1. Spread your legs apart as far as possible into a wide V.

2.   Pull your legs together quickly.

3.   Pull your knees up to your chin (without pushing your chin forward).

4.   Straighten your legs to starting position and repeat rapidly for one minute.

Do other variations of this exercise while you lie on your back by rapidly crossing one straightened leg over the other one or by doing a forward and then a backward bicycling motion. Other exercises you have done by grasping the side of the pool or the gutter may be done away from the pool wall by using kickboards.

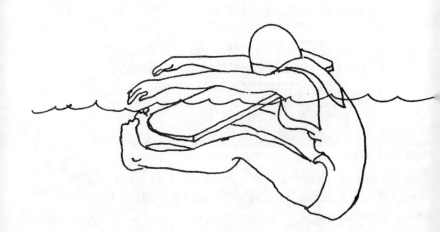

BEAVER TAIL

Starting Position

Lie on your back and hold the pool gutter behind you. Place a kickboard between your thighs so that most of the large part of the board protrudes upward.

Movement

1. As you keep the upper part of your body immobile, vigorously swing from your waist and hips so that you flip the board from side to side. The board acts like a paddle that resists the water; so it should alternately smack the water; right (under); up and over; left (under); up and over, etc. This must be done very rapidly for thirty seconds to one minute.

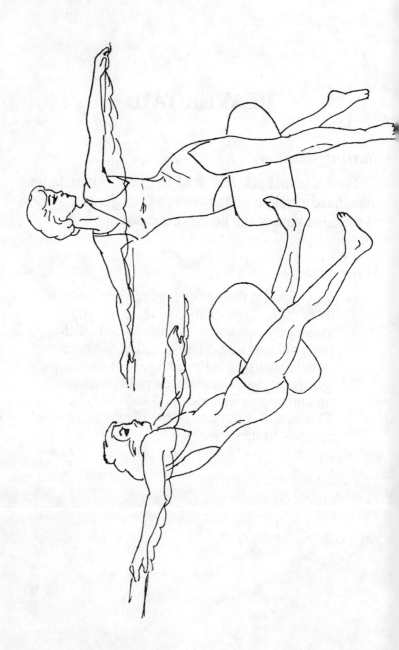

BOARD WALK

Starting Position

This exercise should be done in water slightly over your head or in water that is deep enough not to permit your toes to touch the bottom. Stand erect in the water, supported by kickboards under each arm. Maintain the erect position throughout execution of the exercise.

Movement

1. Move your legs from the hip to the toe by making very large steps in the water. Keep your legs straight. Your legs should move as swiftly as possible like a stiff-legged doll. Do this for one minute.

Variations

Keeping the above position, being certain that you are vertical in the water, practice a fast flutter kick. Practice a frog kick, the breast stroke kick (whip kick), the egg-beater kick, and the scissors kick. Also simply tread water.

Explanation

Although you should stay in the same spot, you likely will move some through the water. It is important to keep your body erect and your feet directly below your torso. If you do not know how to swim, do not do this exercise in water that is over your head unless you are closely guarded. This exercise and its variations may be done without kickboards. When you become expert, do the exercise with both hands above the water.

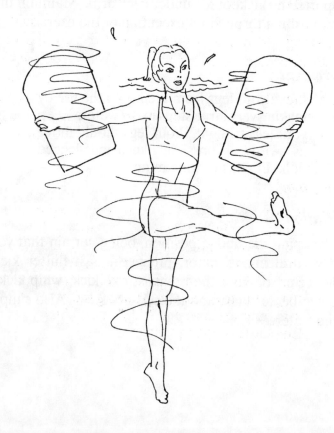

BOARD-BOATING

Starting Position

You may do this exercise in any depth of water. Position the kickboard under your legs so that you are sitting on it. Hold the board lightly with both hands at each end of the board and place the board underneath part of your thighs. Balance the board as you would sit in a swing. You may need to experiment to find your center of balance -- either forward toward the back of your knees, or backward toward your fanny. The kickboard should be perpendicular to your lower legs and you should be in a sitting position, your back very straight. Keep your arms under the water's surface.

Movement

1. Slowly let go of the board to free your arms. Straighten both arms directly in front of you, and keep your arms and your shoulders under the water's surface. Spread your arms apart until they are stright out to sides. Keep pulling the water with your arms as you "ride" your "chair." Emphasis is upon pulling.

Explanation

Move forward for fifteen to twenty yards. Without losing your balance or getting off the kickboard, reverse and move backward for the same distance This exercise is excellent for firming your upper arms and chest and also for developing and maintaining balance. You may simply sit on the board and move both your arms at the same time, making very large circles so that your arms are underwater and they also swing up and over the surface.

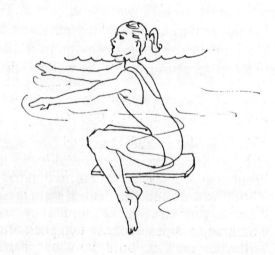

SHOOT-THROUGHS

Starting Position

Lie flat on your back on the surface of the water, legs together and relaxed. Both arms should be supported by kickboards so that your body forms a cross. Give yourself space from the wall and from other people. Your feet are straight ahead of you.

Movements

1. Pull your fanny down and your knees up to your chin in a sitting position. At the same time, push your head and arms forward. Tilt your whole body into a prone, stomach position. Your legs now are straight behind you, toes pointed.

2. You will move from a prone stomach position to a prone back position again by pulling your knees under your body and shoulders back as you thrust your pointed toes forward.

3. Continue to alternate these two positions as fast as you can until you have done the cycle of two positions ten times.

Variation

Another version of the same exercise is to spread your legs into a straddle splits position as you change from moving forward to backward and vice versa. For example, as you lie on your back and begin to change to the stomach position, you spread your legs. When your legs are below you, they are spread to their widest position and you are sitting up. As your legs circle to your rear, they come together as you finally lie on your stomach. Try alternating closed and opened leg shoot-throughs.

Explanation

This is a great back and body relaxer that may be done with or without kickboards, fast or slowly.

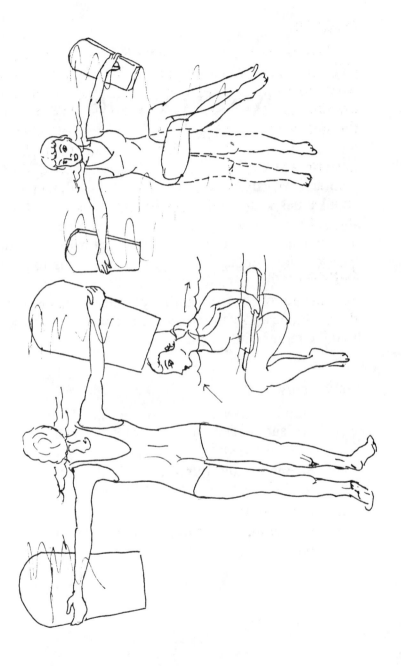

WING FLAPPERS

Starting Position

Stand away from the wall in at least chest deep water. At all times keep your shoulders submerged. It may help to spread your legs into a large Y in order to keep your balance. Place a kickboard lengthwise (if your arms are long enough) from your underarms to your fingertips. You may prefer to hold the board crosswise (see illustration). Also, you may want to exercise one arm at a time and stand beside the pool wall so you can hold the gutter with one hand.

Movements

1. Stand in the water so that your shoulders are submerged and so your arms are straight out and lying on top of the water.

2. Strongly pull your arms and the kickboards straight down to your sides.

1. Let your arms and the boards rise to the surface and again repeat the downward pull.

Explanation

If you cannot keep your balance and/or your feet on the bottom as you exercise both arms at the same time, exercise one arm at a time and hold to the pool gutter with the free arm. Switch arms and be sure to exercise them both. This exercise is most effective if you use kickboards; however, it is also good if you do it without the boards.

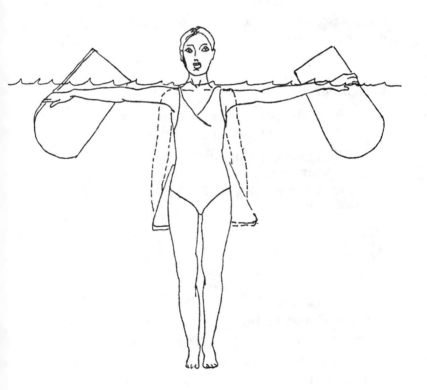

RUB-A-DUB-DUB

Starting Position

Stand straight in shoulder deep water, or squat in more shallow water so that your shoulders are under the surface at all times. Keep your back straight throughout the exercise. Hold a kickboard by each of its ends, lengthwise, so that the board is across your chest and close to your body.

Movements

1. Push the board very hard until your arms are straight down in the water.

2. Pull the board up quickly to the top of the water again. Repeat these two movements as fast as possible for sixty seconds.

Explanation

These two movements should be made as fast as possible; however, each time the board is pushed down, your arms must be fully straightened. The movements resemble clothes scrubbing on an old-fashioned board. Keep your back straight and try to keep your feet on the bottom of the pool. This is a strenuous exercise if it is done quickly and with effort. It is ineffective out of the water because it is the resistance of the water that creates the challenge. It strengthens shoulders and it firms the upper arms. After you become proficient, use two or three boards stacked on top of each other to increase the necessary effort.

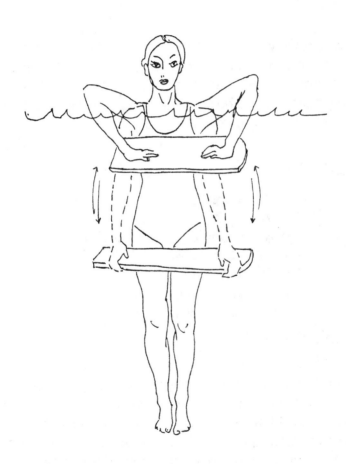

KICKBOARD LEG LIFTS

Starting Position

Stand with your back close to the pool wall, your arms extended along the gutter or however they are comfortable. Place a kickboard between your legs near the area of the knees or a little lower. For best results the board should be perpendicular, or parallel with your legs. It helps to maintain the position of the board if you cross your ankles. Otherwise, the board may pop up suddenly.

Movements

1. Permit the board and your legs to float to the surface of the water. Keep your back against the side of the pool.

2. As you keep your shoulders and back against the pool wall, pull your legs with the board downward through the water so that your heels hit the pool wall at the bottom.

3. Permit the board and your legs to surface again, and again force them back down through the water. Repeat this ten times.

4. Keeping the board between your legs, turn over on your tummy so that you face

the pool wall. Hold the gutter with both hands. Let the board and your legs rise to the surface so that you are lying prone.

5. Pull your legs and the board through the water so that your toes touch the pool wall. On both your back and on your stomach, your stomach muscles, not your arms or back, should force your legs downward. Your legs should be like a pendulum that swings from the surface of the water in an arc to the pool wall. Repeat the exercise on your stomach ten times.

Explanation

For most people, this exercise is very difficult (especially when they do it on the back) at first. This takes practice. Movements should originate from the waist and the pelvic/hip area. It is a tummy flattener. If you have trouble doing this exercise, try doing it without the kickboard. Later use a pull-buoy between your legs; graduate to the kickboard.

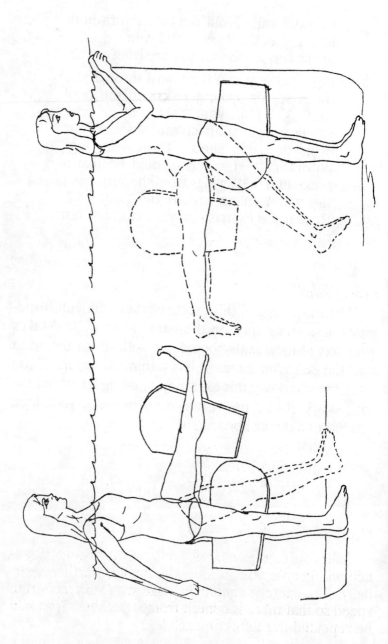

POOL WALL SPLITS

Starting Position

Face the pool wall and hold the gutter with both hands, arms' length, between your legs. Spread your legs far apart in a splits position. The feet are flat against the wall and high -- just below the hands.

Movements

1. Flatten your left foot on the wall as you bend the left knee over the foot and straighten the right leg at the same time. Move your hands along the gutter as you do the movement.

2. Reverse by straightening the left leg and bending the right knee over the right foot.

3. Alternate these above positions, swinging back and forth without changing the position of your feet.

Explanation

Like most stretches, this is a slow movement. Practice will enable you to spread your legs farther apart daily. The exercise should be performed with moderate speed so that there is benefit from stretching. It should be repeated five times on each leg.

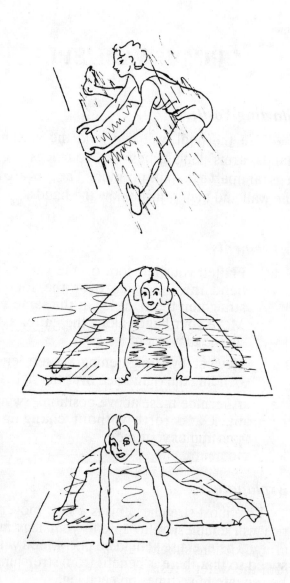

SPLITS WALL WALK

Starting Position

This starting position and the position you will maintain is almost the same as that of the Pool Wall Splits. Both hands hold the pool gutter between the spread legs; however, the feet do not have to be kept flat against the side of the pool.

Movements

1. Pull your legs together and then repeatedly spread them as you walk against the poolside. Your hands and feet both will walk at the same time. Move swiftly in one direction, e.g., the right.

2. Reverse your direction and walk your feet and hands against the poolside, e.g., the left. Continue to reverse your directions from right to left after you have gained momentum in the one direction.

Explanation

This exercise should be done very fast and the reversal of directions should be swift in order to get the benefit from the water's resistance. Vary the number of steps you take from side to side. Lower the number of steps and increase the number of reversals as you continue to exercise for about sixty seconds.

PRECAUTIONARY POINTS

General
Causes of Beginners' Blues

1. *Lack of self-confidence*
2. *Self-consciousness*
3. *Impatience*
4. *Insufficient warm-up*
5. *Overly exaggerated movements*
6. *Lack of kinesthetic awareness*
7. *Unrealistic -- or no -- goals*
8. *Self-indulgence excusing difficult efforts*
9. *Forcing movements that are too painful*
10. *Lack of perseverance*
11. *Ignorance of or ignoring medical and expert advice*

BASIC POINTS TO REMEMBER

1. Include adequate warm-ups and cool-offs during every session, especially during aerobic inclusion sessions. Warm-ups are necessary for the muscles to maintain strenuous movements with safety. Cool-downs help to gradually decrease the blood flow throughout the whole body without danger of cutting circulation off from some parts of the body. Always cool down before showering. Do not take a hot or cold shower; take a tepid shower.

2. Stretch muscles adequately and properly when you start each exercise session. This prevents cramps and it reduces muscle soreness.

3. Establish and maintain an appropriate fitness level by exercising a minimum of three times a week for a minimum of thirty minutes of continuous movements after warm-ups and cool-downs.

4. Regulate breathing in order to achieve utilization of oxygen and to prevent fatigue.

5. Gradually re-establish activity to prevent further injury -- and to increase muscle tone -- to weak or injured areas.

6. Maintain good posture throughout an exercise session as well as during other activities. Bad posture can result in stress or even injury.

7. If an exercise or a movement creates pain or stress that is not a natural result of unaccustomed effort, change the movements or replace that exercise with another one.

8. Prevent   dehydration by drinking water immediately after -- even during -- a session.

9. Exercising is a part of your health program. It cannot create miracles. Police your diet carefully and do not eat heavily after a session or at any other time. Stop eating before you are satisfied. One fringe benefit of regular and adequate exercise is reduction of appetite.

10. Know your body and listen "to what it tells you." Periodically take your pulse during exercise sessions as well as at other times. Learn to take the pulse easily and properly.

AEROBICS

Non-stop activity should last a minimum of thirty to forty-five minutes. You must maintain your target heart rate. To be on the safe side, check your heart rate approximately every five minutes. Exercises in this section should be done very rapidly without pauses between exercises. Use music of a fast tempo, some moderate tempo, but all with a definite beat.

There are two main kinds of strenuous exercise, aerobic and anaerobic. Though both kinds benefit tone and strengthen the muscles, aerobics benefits the cardio-vascular system.

Anaerobics usually are calisthenics or sprinting; aerobics are distance workouts or intervals. Anaerobics break down carbohydrates, the energy source. Aerobics break down carbohydrates, protein and fats. Anaerobics produce the by-product, lactic acid, that causes muscle fatigue and soreness; whereas, aerobics are more efficient for they demand efficient use of heart and lungs with by-products of carbon-dioxide and water. Although anaerobics make demands for oxygen, they do not do so for sufficient time to be of value to the heart and lungs.

On the other hand, aerobics increase cardiovascular fitness and muscle metabolism. Anaerobics is not a sustainable energy source, but aerobics is a sustainable energy source.

Doubtless Kenneth H. Cooper* coined the word, *aerobics*; he certainly has made it popular. He has eloquently defined aerobics and he maintains that exercise must be hard enough to create a sustained heartbeat of 150 beats per minute in order to get the training effects and benefits from the activity. He points out that the real effect of such exercise begins about five minutes after you start exercising (at training rate) and that the benefit continues so long as you keep up that rate. One can exercise at a somewhat lower heart rate that demands much oxygen intake, but you have to continue that exercise longer than five minutes. In other words, if you are breathing very hard and if your pulse rate is about 150 beats per minute, you likely are getting some aerobic exercise.

Exercises for conditioning and strength and even the warm-ups and taper-offs in this book can be used aerobically if you exercise fast, hard, and continuously. You must keep moving from one exercise to another without any pause -- that is if you want to condition your heart and lungs to get oxygen to your tissues for calories to

---

*Kenneth H. Cooper, *Aerobics* (N.Y.: A Bantam Book, published by arrangement with M. Evans & Co., Inc., 1968), p. 25.

---

ourn rapidly. Exercise must be rhythmic and it must involve your whole body.

You must constantly ask yourself, "Honestly, how hard am I working?" This is not always an easily answered question. Not only must you stop rationalizing your laziness, but you must find the appropriate intensity of exertion for yourself. This level must not be too strenuous -- nor too lenient. This happy medium is mostly determined by finding your normal and your training heart rates (see introduction to this text). Generally speaking, people who sustain sixty to eighty percent of their maximum aerobic power will have a heartbeat that is seventy to eighty-five percent of their maximum heart rate.

Of course, heart rates vary with every individual. The lower your resting heart rate and the quicker your heart rate drops to your resting rate after performing aerobics, or strenuous exercise, the more cardiovascularly fit you are. Periodic (every five to ten minutes) pulse check while you are exercising helps to reveal your rate of improvement and if you are overly exerting yourself.

You must begin by knowing your resting heart rate, ideally, before you arise in the morning or always after you have been quietly sitting for at least fifteen minutes. Your resting heart rate is the number of times your heart beats per minute while you are at rest.

On the other hand, your working heart rate that you take during exercising may be quickly done by counting your pulse for six seconds and multiplying by ten. While you take your working heart rate keep moving slowly. Stay within your working heart rate range and never exceed your maximum rate. Those who are beginning exercises should keep their rate below 140 -- at least for the first two weeks.

It is vital to monitor your recovery heart rate, that is, the heart rate that drops after doing strenuous exercise. Take your pulse five minutes after the aerobic exercises. Your pulse should be below 120. Take your pulse rate ten minutes later. It should be below 100. If your pulse is higher than these figures, cut back on the intensity of your movements. While you take your recovery heart rate, continue to move slowly in the water.

The following is a general guide for aerobic training heart rate zones. The first column is the age. The second column is for people who have a history of heart problems; so they should not exceed this rate unless they are under the direction of their physician. It is based on seventy percent maximum attainable heart rate.

The third column lists the desired heart rate for normally healthy people, or equal to eighty percent maximum attainable heart rate. The fourth column should be used only by athletes who are in good condition. It lists the eighty-five percent maximum attainable heart rate.

AGE	HEART PATIENTS	NORMALLY HEALTHY	ADVANCED ATHLETE
20	140	160	170
25	136	156	166
30	133	152	161
35	129	148	157
40	126	144	153
45	122	140	149
50	119	136	144
55	115	132	140
60	112	128	136
70	105	120	127

Most authorities recommend that average people exercise fifteen to thirty minutes of target-range exercises for three or four times a week. This, of course, is preceded and followed by five to ten minutes warm-up and five to ten minutes taper-off. The total exercise period (minimum) is thus thirty minutes plus twenty minutes, or about fifty minutes to an hour of three to four exercise periods per week.

You must work the whole time during your session to keep your working heart rate at its appropriate pace. Lollygagging, conversation at the end of the pool or while you leisurely side stroke, simply do not count.

On the other hand, you should exercise for the sheer joy of moving around and playing instead of punching a hand-held calculator or making business or work of water exercises. Ballpark figures are necessary for safety and for basic organization, but these figures have a way of becoming ends in themselves instead of a means to an end. It is a mystery why children have so much fun skipping rope and adults make hard work of it. Why do children jump into water and play exuberant tag, and ladies and gentlemen float with dry hair like indifferent lily pads?

Adults have learned some negative things, such as fear and inhibited self-consciousness. Some are afraid to exercise; afraid to jazz up their heartbeat. Women may not want to be seen with wet hair. Too many people discover that exercise with any aerobic value at all makes them out of breath, and that's uncomfortable. So they rationalize and even say that their physicians have told them not to exert themselves. If this is the case these people belong in a hospital, not in a swimming pool.

Usually people are not at all allergic to chlorine. The reason the water makes their eyes sting is that people do not usually open their eyes under water. Stinging usually is caused by the action of chlorine oxidizing impurities in the water -- not by chlorine itself. If this troubles you, use a pair of swimming goggles, never a mask, for a mask inhibits proper movements.

You will postpone your visit to the hospital or to the grave if you participate in aerobic exercises that you sensibly adapt to your personal limitations and your potential. Your circulatory-respiratory (CR) endurance is the basis of your work capacity. Muscles need oxygen in order to release energy you have consumed as food. For average strong muscles, the biggest limitation is the rate at which muscles receive oxygen. This rate of receiving oxygen is determined by the size of your lungs, by the time it takes for the blood to deliver oxygen to the muscles, and by the time it takes for the muscles to get rid of metabolic waste. Obviously, the cardiovascular system's endurance and fitness depends upon the efficiency of your lungs. Strong and enduring muscles are needed for any activity that can cause maximum changes in the CR rate. It is the problem of the chicken and the egg. Your CR fitness is measured by the number of heartbeats per minute. The more efficient your CR system, the less hard it has to work as you exercise, and the faster it can return to a normal beat after you exercise. From this point of view, it is not so important how many repetitions of an exercise you do, but how many repetitions you perform in a specific time period.

Performing fast repetitions of a movement or moving in the water, requires special effort and knowledge of breathing. There is an old saying, "Oh, that's as easy as breathing!" Like everything else in life, especially in doing exercises or swimming, there is a right and a wrong way even to breathe. Breathing is not as simple as some people would like to think. In fact, the most important thing to learn and the first thing that should be taught in swimming is the proper way to breathe. I have seen many heads-up and badly rolling swimmers who would have been fairly good swimmers if only they had learned how to breathe. Some people even go so far as to use a mask and snorkel to swim laps because they never learned how to rhythmically breathe while they swam. Whether you are exercising in or out of the water, you need to practice rhythmic breathing.

In order to learn how to rhythmically breathe, follow these simple steps:

1. Stand in waist deep water with one leg placed behind the other in a giant stepping position. Lean your body and head over the water and hold on to the side of the pool with one hand. The other hand and arm should dangle at your side.

2. Take a breath and place your face on the surface of the water, just to the hairline. Cover your face, especially your eyes, but not your whole head. Hold your breath for at least the count of two. Bubble out the air in steady streams from your nose and your mouth.

3. As you finish bubbling out the air, slowly but deliberately turn your head and one side of your face and ear towards your extended, resting, arm. Do not lift your head from the water. This is the major error. Simply turn your head so that one ear and one cheek are still in the water, and inhale new air. Be sure to open your mouth wide and breathe in through your mouth only -- not your nose.

4. Rotate your face so that it again is looking downward to the bottom of the pool, and your eyes are under water. Again, exhale the air steadily from both the nose and the mouth.

Repeat the above steps until you can easily rotate your face from your eyes being covered by water to one ear's being submerged. Do this rhythmically fifty to a hundred times. As you practice, do not stop to wipe water from your eyes or your face; they will just get wet again anyhow. To practice breath holding, simply inhale, turn your face into the water, and exhale under the water when you no longer can hold your breath. You should practice rhythmic breathing first on one side only after you discover which is your more comfortable side. Later learn to rhythmically breathe on both sides. Start by doing your cycle of breathing for five, then for ten or twenty counts without stopping.

Just after you inhale and put your mouth underwater, begin to exhale in a steady trickle from both your nose and mouth. If you exhale only from your mouth, you may get water up your nose, and that is uncomfortable. Later when you become skilled, try explosive breathing; however, many experts disagree about this. At any rate, hold your breath for a couple of seconds and suddenly explode out almost all the air. Save a little air to exhale in order to clear the water away from your mouth as you turn your head to one side in order to inhale again.

Practice rhythmic breathing while you hold to the side of the pool and flutter kick. You also may practice this breathing while you use a kickboard or while you bob or move in the water.

For the sake of safety and security, take at least one swimming lesson and inform the guard or instructor that you want to learn how to breathe properly in the water. Engage an American Red Cross Beginning Swim Instructor (BSI) or Water Safety Instructor (WSI) if you really want correct and safe help.

Exhaling against the pressure of water gives your lungs much more exercise than simply breathing out air into air; another great advantage of swimming and water exercises. Not only is it necessary to know how to breathe properly in the water, it also is necessary to know proper breathing in doing land exercises, especially jumping rope, weight lifting, jogging, gymnastics, ballet and any other exercise that "gets you out of breath." It is generally agreed that the most valuable exercise does get you winded. If it does not, you simply are not working hard enough.

KNEE-KNOCKERS

Starting Position

Stand in waist or chest deep water away from the wall. Fold your fingers behind your head or neck, elbows straight out in opposite directions.

Movements

1. Quickly twist your body as you pull up your left knee to touch your right elbow.

2. Quickly twist your body as you pull up your right knee to touch your left elbow. Alternate touching elbows to opposite knees for a minute or at least thirty seconds each.

Variations

Bend the right side and hit the right elbow with the right knee and visa versa. Hop with the legs spread frog fashion. Repeat this for thirty seconds.

Next, bend so that you hit your left elbow to your left ankle and vice versa. You need to bend more for this one than for any of the others; also, you need to spread your knees more for this exercise than you do for the others.

Explanation

As soon as you are accustomed to doing this exercise, alternate it with the variations and perform them as fast as possible for a minimum of one minute.

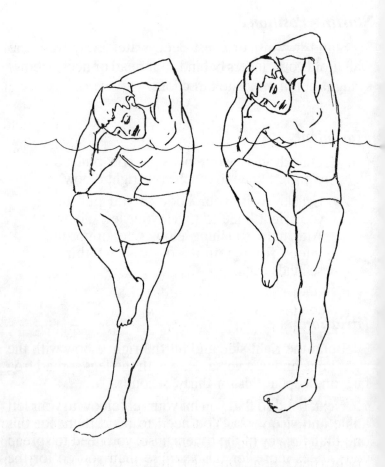

JUMPING JACKS

Starting Position

Stand erect in at least waist deep water. Your arms should be at your sides and your feet should be together, This exercise may be done so that your arms come out of the water if you are in waist depth, or so that your arms come only to the surface of the water if you stand in neck deep water. The latter is the more challenging,

Movements

1. Jump with your feet wide apart. At the same time swing your arms high above your head so that your hands touch.

2. Jump so that your feet are together and your hands and arms hit the tip of the water or come down to your sides. Continue these movements for a minimum of thirty seconds or fifty jumps.

Variations

Keeping your back straight, jump and change your foot position so that the back leg is straight and the front right knee is bent. One leg is in front of the other. Jump and reverse your foot position so that the back leg is forward with the knee bent and the front leg is straight behind you. Your hands and arms will swing over your head, one in front of you and one behind you in opposition to your foot position. Every time the legs change position, the arms change position.

Explanation

In both variations the legs and arms change at the same time and quickly. The whole point of the exercise is to execute it as fast as you can with hops between the positions.

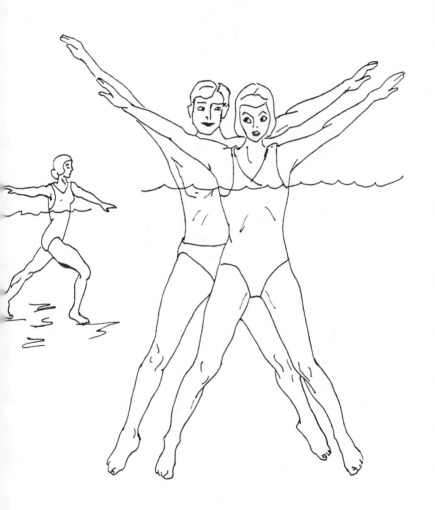

TOE-TOUCHES

Starting Position

Stand straight; look forward with your arms at your sides in waist to chest deep water.

Movements

1. Jump as high as possible, moving your feet to the surface of the water and your legs spread far apart. Try to touch the left fingers to the left toes and the right fingers to the right toes. Keep the legs straight.

2. Return to starting position between jumps. Do at least twenty jumps without any pause.

3. Alternate the touching so that you raise the leg and bring the right hand to the left toes as you extend the left arm behind you. Reverse and touch the left fingers to the right toes.

4. Jump and touch fingers of both hands to the right toe. Return to starting position and then reverse by extending the arms and touching the fingers of both hands to the left toes.

Explanation

The torso will have to be bent to do these movements. Keep your arms and your legs very straight. When you do number one, bending your knees just before taking a high jump may help you get elevation. Both feet should leave the pool bottom at exactly the same time, and both arms should be extended at the same time. Aim to get the toes to the top of the water and then to raise them above the water. Both one and two should be done with fast hops between movements. Parts three and four of this exercise should be done very rapidly.

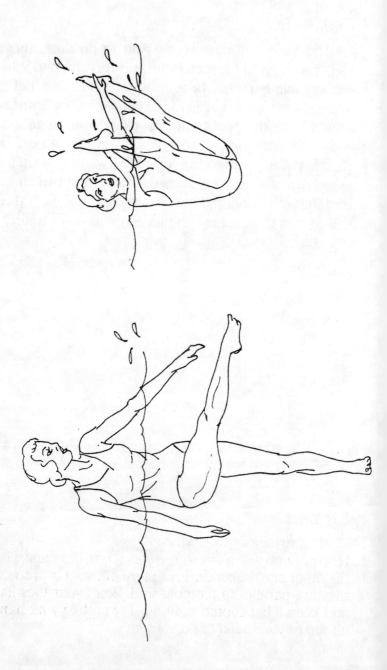

FROG JUMP

Starting Position

Stand erect, facing the pool wall and lightly holding both hands on the gutter, your feet a few inches apart and your body is a few inches from the wall. This exercise also may be done away from the wall, in the pool area.

Movements

1. Quickly jump so that one knee bends and breaks the water's surface.

2. Quickly jump on the working foot now so that the other knee bends and breaks the water's surface. Try to straighten the supporting leg each time. Do this exercise for a minimum of thirty seconds. Count the number of times you jump and try to increase the number each time.

Explanation

The virtue of this exercise is that it is done very fast. Hop or jump when one foot leaves the bottom and when the other one descends. Try to turn out your hips so that they are parallel to the pool wall. Point your toes hard and keep a bat-footed position. Try putting your hands on top of your head or on your hips.

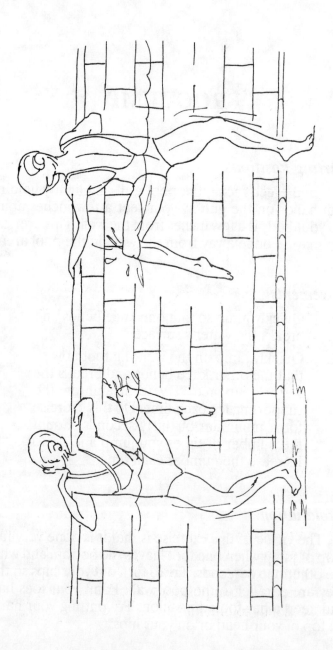

IN-OUTS

Starting Position

Stand with your arms at your sides and away from the side of the pool in chest deep or waist deep water.

Movements

1. With both legs at exactly the same time, jump up high. Your knees should be bent so that you are in a ball. At the same time straighten your arms between your legs so that both hands touch the heels of both feet at the same time.

2. Jump back to standing position.

3. Jump up quickly in the same fashion, but this time straighten your arms so that they are outside your bent legs. Touch your heels.

4. Recover to starting position, then alternately straighten your arms inside and then outside your legs. Continue to jump very hard and fast as the arms alternate their positions. Do this for thirty seconds to one minute.

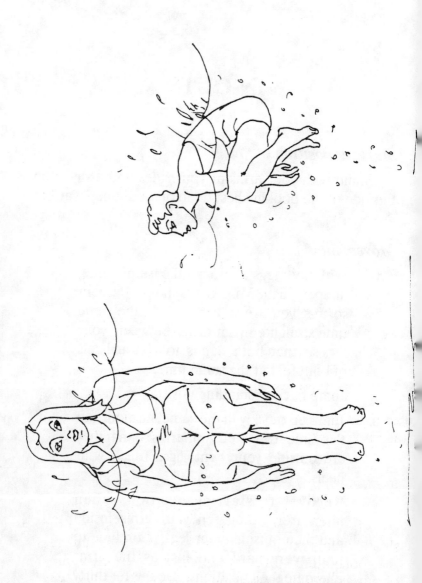

LEG EXCHANGE

Starting Position

Stand facing the wall and holding the gutter with both hands. Keep your back straight and look straight ahead. Stand on one leg and extend the other leg directly behind you. Keep your shoulders parallel to the pool wall.

Movement

Hop quickly from leg to leg with one straight leg supporting you and the other straight leg extending behind you. Continue to exchange the positions of your legs very fast for at least thirty seconds. Count the number of times one foot hits the pool bottom. Do another exercise and then do this one again. Count again; see if you can increase the number of exchanges.

Explanation

Do this exercise in thirty second intervals with fifteen seconds between them. The heel of the extended foot should break water and the supporting foot should press the pool bottom with every exchange. Count the number of times one foot presses the bottom and try to increase the number during each interval. Keep both legs straight at all times. Arch the back to keep your torso erect.

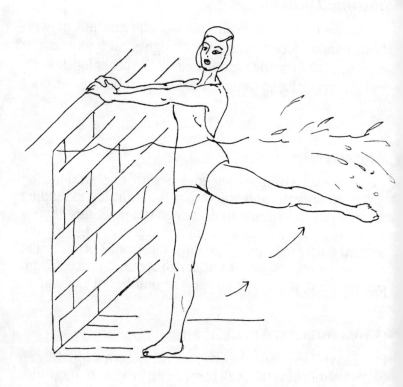

LEG SWING JUMP

Starting Position

Stand in waist or shoulder depth water away from the side of the pool.

Movements

1. Swing your right leg out at least hip high, directly to your right side while you jump on your left leg.

2. Swiftly swing your left leg out to your left side as your right leg and foot come down.

3. Repeat this set of movements for one minute.

Explanation

Thrust your legs out and up against the water very fast so that you get out of breath. Think of a clock's pendulum and of your legs swinging like that pendulum as you quickly cross the pool. Exercise your feet and ankles by pointing your toes every time they leave the pool bottom. You may keep your arms above you with very straight back or you may want to hold a ball between your hands above you. As your right leg swings to the water's surface, bend hard towards that leg and vice versa. The hard bending from side to side will add extra waist exercise movement.

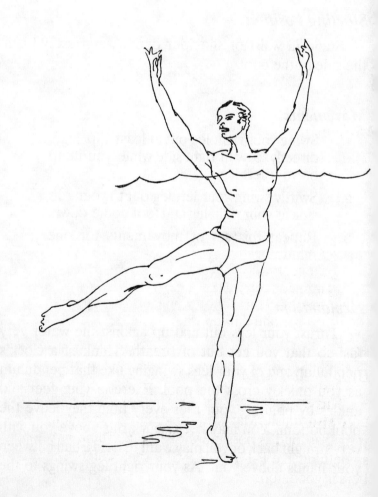

1-2-3 JUMP

Starting Position

Stand straight, away from the pool wall, in waist to chest deep water. Your arms hang by your sides. Keep your feet and legs together.

Movements

1. Throw your arms straight over your head as you begin and as you continue to do this exercise. Make two jumps, each time reaching for the roof.

2. The third jump should be the biggest -- try to reach all the way out of the water.

3. Repeat: one or two smaller jumps; then immediately make a huge, out of water leap. Do this set of movements ten times or for one minute.

Explanation

The exercise must be done very fast with no stops until you finish. Maximum benefit can be attained by yelling as loud as possible with each big jump or spelling something like F-I-T-N-E-S-S! Simply yelling out numbers is good, too.

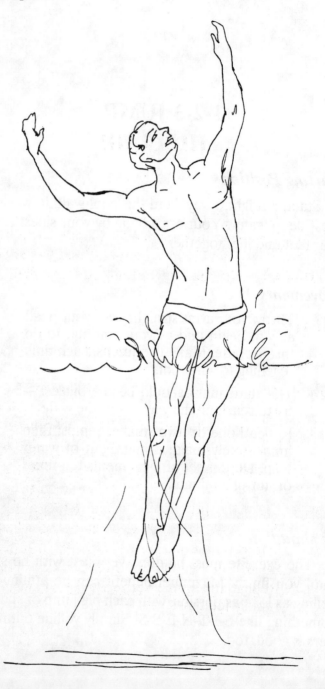

HURRAH!

Starting Position

Stand straight in shoulder deep water. Close your fists and bend your elbows. Be sure the elbows are close to your sides with the fists touching your shoulders.

Movements

1. Thrust the right arm straight overhead -- to the sky.

2. Bring the right arm back to the shoulder with elbow bent.

3. Thrust the left arm overhead and recover it in the same way.

4. Thrust both arms to your sides and open the fists.

5. Close the fists and bend the elbows up close to the sides and close the fists.

6. Thrust both arms hard above the head; recover to bent elbow position.

7. Repeat the whole series of movements rapidly ten times.

Explanation

In or out of the water, this exercise must be done with much gusto and force for it to have any value at all. Opening and closing fists under water is a good hand exercise if it also is done so that all fingers stretch and so that the fists are very tight. This exercise also may be done with straight arms. First you thrust one arm high in the air with the other one lowered; then you reverse the movement. Next you throw both arms straight up. Making a fist gives more force to your movements. Do this exercise by jumping or leaping high each time you thrust up an arm or both arms.

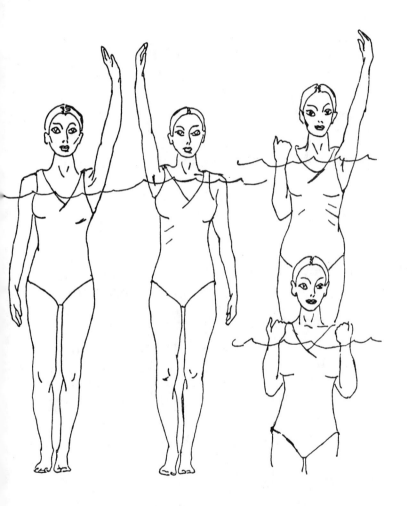

FLUTTER-FAST

Starting Position

Lie flat on your tummy, holding the gutter with both hands and legs straight on top of the water behind you.

Movements

1. As fast as you can, do the crawl stroke flutter kick on your stomach. Accelerate your speed as you kick. The movement should originate from your hips, not from your knees. Legs should have a waving motion, not stiff, but straight.

2. Turn onto your back and do the same thing. Grasp the gutter near your ears. This kick will have a heavy upbeat; whereas, the stomach kick had a heavy downbeat.

3. Lie on your right side and hold the side of the pool with the left hand braced on top of the pool wall. Flutter your legs by pulling them quickly together and apart; then flutter again back and forth.

4. Reverse sides; lie on your left side and hold the side of the pool with your right hand braced against the pool wall. Flutter

your legs; pull them quickly together and
apart.

Explanation

The flutter kick should be done not too deeply and
very fast. The movements must originate from the hips
and not from the knees; however, the legs should not be
stiff. Try to achieve a strong yet a waving motion. While
you are swimming the crawl stroke, you should not splash
or let the instep (the top of the foot) break water. Only
the heels of the feet should slightly break water. While
you do this exercise, however, kick hard enough so that
the whole foot breaks water. You may alternate speeds
of fluttering for all four positions, but each movement
should be done for a minimum of thirty seconds. Avoid
a pumping, a cycling motion, or just bending the knees
excessively.

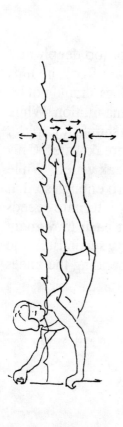

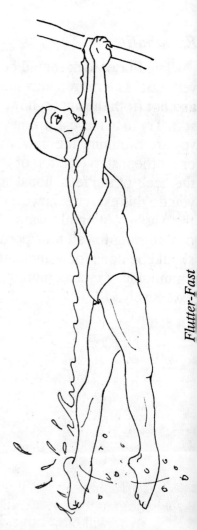

Flutter-Fast

BOBBING

Starting Position

If you can swim, do this exercise in water that is two to three feet over your head. If you cannot swim, you can do this exercise in chest deep water. Take a deep breath. Stand straight with your hands turned toward your thighs and your arms straight.

Movements

1. As you submerge into a squat, feet on the bottom and legs in a frog-like position, throw your arms up vertically, straight above your head.

2. Quickly and powerfully straighten your legs (together) and push hard from the pool bottom. At the same time pull your straight arms directly down to your sides. At this point exhale, and explode straight up and out of the water.

3. As you regain standing position, repeat the above movements. When your head is out of the water take in a deep breath that you will blow out as you again emerge to the surface.

Explanation

All bobbing should be powerfully done. You should blast out of the water and expose your body to the hips. Bobbing develops leg and breath power. It helps shoulders and arms, and it produces heavy, forced breathing. The motion should be repeated in a rhythmical and vigorous series with no interruptions or stopping. You may bob in one place or you may travel in any desired direction.

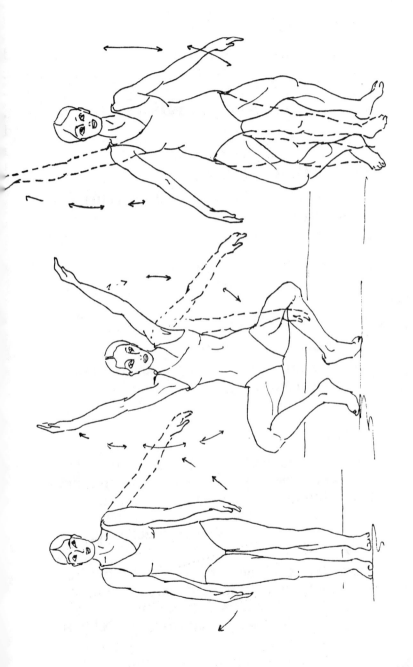

MULE KICK

Starting Position

Face the pool wall and hold the gutter with both hands. Place both feet flat up against the wall of the pool about a foot below your hands. Your back is hunched.

Movements

1. Violently push both feet out from the wall and without touching the bottom extend your legs behind you.

2. Return to starting position and repeat the movement.

Variations

1. As you push both feet away from the poolside, you spread your feet in a kind of splits position so that your feet make a circle until they meet again behind you. You may reverse the direction of the circles.

2. Turn one side to the pool wall, both feet below your hand. If you are lying on your right side you will hold to the wall with your right hand. The left hand will rest

on your left hip. Push violently away from the wall and extend your legs out to the side. Reverse this and turn onto the left side and do the same thing. Whether you do a plain mule kick, a circling leg mule kick, or a side kick, be sure that you do the exercise very fast and powerfully. Count the times you do the kicks in thirty seconds and try to better your score.

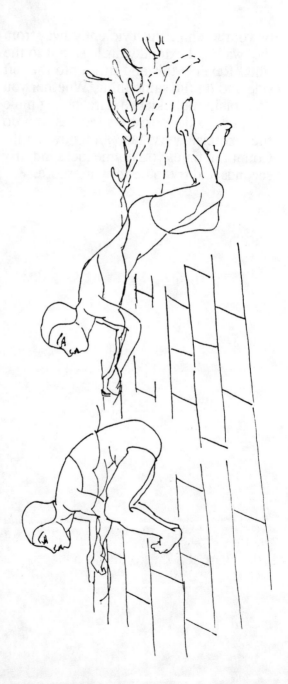

KNEE FAN

Starting Position

Stand in chest deep water. Keep your torso erect and bend your knees in right angles.

Movements

1. Spread your bent knees as far apart as possible, exposing the insides of your legs.

2. Quickly pull your knees and legs together so that they are closed in front of you, but they still are bent.

3. Spread your bent knees again as far apart as possible.

Explanation

Beginning at a moderate speed flop your knees and legs together and then apart. Increase your speed and repeat the exercise for forty-five seconds to one minute.

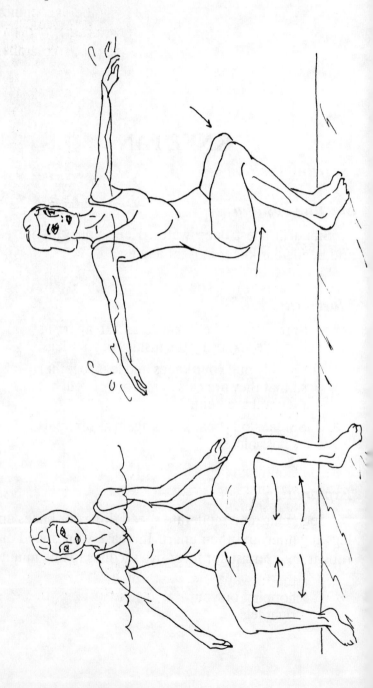

KARATE KICK

Starting Position

Stand in waist deep water away from the pool's side.

Movements

1. Stand on your right leg. Pull up your left knee and keeping your leg elevated quickly kick and straighten the leg as if you were violently kicking a door or some object. Remain erect. Keep kicking hard without lowering the working leg for a minimum of ten kicks.

2. Without lowering the working leg, continue to kick hard, only you kick directly out to the side. Do a minimum of ten hard and fast kicks.

3. Continuing to kick without lowering the working leg, kick to the rear. You will bend and straighten the leg hard as you did in the other positions, for a minimum of ten times.

4. Reverse the exercise by doing the kicks in the forward, side, and back positions by hopping on your left leg and kicking your right leg.

Explanation

With every kick you must hop hard on the supporting leg. Actually, both legs are working hard throughout the exercise. Be sure not to lower the kicking leg at any time. This exercise has intense aerobic potential.

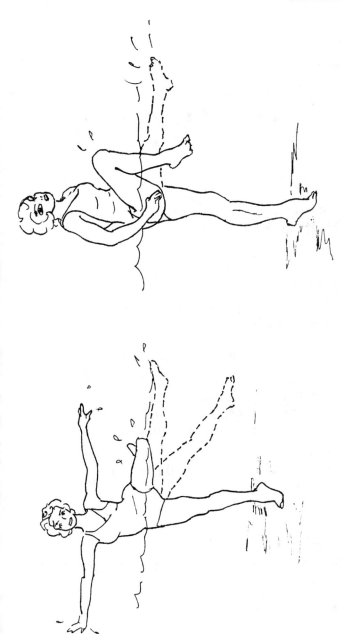

LEG CLAPPERS

Starting Position

Stand in water between chest and shoulder depth away from the side of the pool.

Movements

1. Hop on the right leg and swing the left leg (straight) to the water's surface. At the same time clap both your hands underneath the thigh-knee area.

2. Swiftly swap legs and hop onto the left leg (straight) and swing the right leg to the water's surface. At the same time clap your hands under the thigh-knee area.

3. Continue to quickly swap legs, hopping and kicking upward for thirty to forty-five seconds.

Explanation

This exercise must be done very fast. Work to break the water's surface and to splash with the toes of the kicking leg. Keep both legs straight.

Variation

Jump very hard to make both knees break the water's surface and clap both hands under your bent knees. Repeat a minimum of ten times without any pauses. Bend both knees upward while you jump.

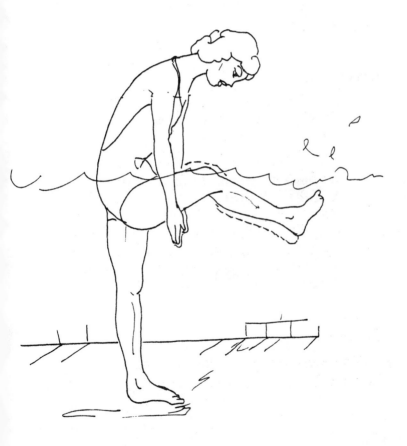

CAN-CAN

Starting Position

Stand erect in waist deep water. You may use your arms as you please.

Movements

1. Jump hard as you pull up the left knee hard towards the surface of the water.

2. Straighten the left leg as it returns to the ground or pool's bottom.

3. Lift the left leg that is straightened, to the surface of the water. Lower the straightened leg to the bottom.

4. Alternate lifting the left leg in bent and in straightened positions at least ten times.

5. Jump hard on the left leg and bend and straighten the right leg -- reverse the exercise.

Explanation

Like other aerobic exercises, this must be done very rapidly. If you do not have a tape or a record to play, think of a circus tune or the Can-Can and move rhythmically.

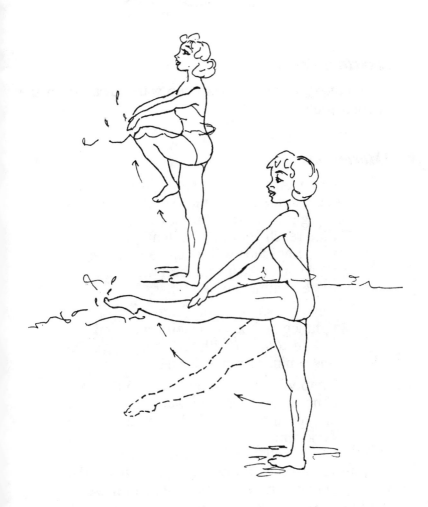

CHARLESTON

Starting Position

Stand straight in waist deep water away from the pool's side.

Movements

1. Jump hard on the left leg while you bend the right knee so that your left foot is straight up to your buttocks. At the same time reach your hand behind you so that your fingertips will touch your toes each time you make a bent, backward kick. Do this a minimum of ten times.

2. Reverse, so that you jump hard on the right leg and bend the left leg behind you as you touch it with your fingertips. Do this a minimum of ten times,

3. Jump very hard on both feet so that you bend both knees downward and the feet are towards the water's surface. At the same time arch your back so that both hands will touch both feet when they surface. Continue to bound from the pool's bottom as you do this exercise at least ten times.

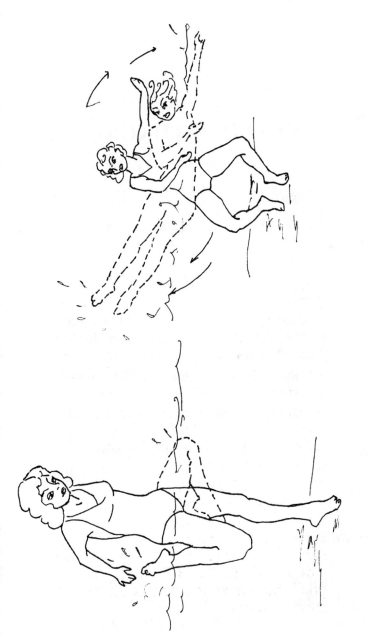

Kremlin Thrust

Charleston

KREMLIN THRUST

Starting Position

Stand erect in waist deep water away from side of the pool.

Movements

1. Bend knees and make both feet leave the bottom at the same time as you thrust your feet to and above the water's surface.

2. As you do number one, stretch your body and arms out to the side, opposite your legs and feet, reaching out in the opposite direction.

3. Regain starting position and repeat the exercise at least five times to the right and then five times to the left.

Explanation

Do only a couple of these exercises on each side to begin; then increase the number as you become increasingly fit. This is an intense exercise and must be done without any pauses between movements or sets.

AEROBIC SETS

The following aerobic exercises may be done in sets, or groups. Select three to four exercises and repeat each of them in succession a minimum of five times each.

ON THE WALL
EXERCISES

1.   **Hop-Skip.** With legs together, kick both of them first to the right and then to the left.

2.   **Twist.** Keep legs together and hop straight up; hop by twisting to the right and then to the left.

3.   **Leg Tuck.** Shoulders against wall; tuck knees, first to the right and then to the left, first on stomach and then on back.

4.   **Double Leg Hop.** Start with legs together, hop up and spread legs apart and then bring them back down together.

5.   **Double Leg Hop II.** Start with legs apart, hop up and pull legs together.

6.   **Double Knee Hop.** Start with straight legs on bottom. Hop and bring bent knees to surface, first to the right and then to the left.

7. **Mule Kick.** Do regular, side kick. Kick one leg at a time; run against the wall. Kick out to sides, coming together behind; then tucking up, semi-circle, full circle -- as in text.

8. **Scissors Kick.** Move legs as scissors, first on one side and then the other.

9. **Flutter Kick.** Stomach, side, back, side, stomach, etc.

10. **Bicycle Kick.** Legs move as if riding a bicycle, first straight, on back and then on each side; alternate left and right.

11. **Breast Stroke Kick.** First on stomach and then on back.

12. **Dolphin Kick.**

13. Alternate all of these by doing the **Frog Jump.**

14. **Leg Exchange.**

AWAY FROM THE WALL
(HOPPING WITH BOTH LEGS)

1. **Frog Jump.**

2. **Jumping Jacks.** Regular; double; forward and back.

3. **Karate Kicks.** Frog, side, back.

4. Jump up and **Flutter Kick.**

5. **Kremlin Thrust.**

6. **Dolphin Kick** as you jump straight up.

7. **Breast Stroke Kick** as you jump straight up.

8. **Leg Clappers.** Single and together.

9. **Leg Cross Hops.** Stand with legs apart, hop up and cross legs.

10. Jump up and twist from one side to the other.

11. Hop, **1-2-3-Hop.**

12. **Hurrah!**

13. Hop and swing arms in a circle.

14. Hop and stretch arms right; hop and stretch arms left.

15. Hop hard and punch arms in and out -- punching bag.

16. Hard jabbing while pulling water with one and then other arm.

17. Rocking horse - one leg forward - rock. Then rock onto back leg. Alternate.

18. Alternate hand to toe touches.

19. Touch both hands to both feet as you jump high.

20. Hop on left leg fully extending right leg (hands touch shoulders, hips, knees, then toes).

21. Hop on one leg making a figure 8 with the other one.

22. **Turkey Wings.** Hop on both legs or run while you flop your elbows. Your hands are on your shoulders and your bent arms are straight out from your shoulders.

FOR GROUPS

SQUARE DANCE ROUTINES

1. High kicks to one side with hands held together in a circle under water.
2. Rip 'n Snort
3. Bend the Line
4. Do-Si-Do
5. Weave the Ring
6. Drive Through
7. Pass Through
8. Texas Star
9. Swing Your Partner
10. Grand Right and Left
11. Alamo
12. Wash Board Run
13. Pass Through

LIFESTYLE

Generally speaking, lifestyles are determined by our values and our personal limitations, physical, psychological, and economic. We who have arthritis, who have diabetes, and who have heart disease or Charcot-Marie Tooth Disease,. etc., have to make very special adjustments in life. More fortunate is everyone else who only has to experience the aging process. Whether we are people approaching puberty or people approaching retirement age, we all have to make a series of adjustments as we move in time from one phase of life into another. We may not even be conscious of modifying our styles of life as we develop -- or adjust.

One of the most common necessities is the adjustment to one of the 109 different types of arthritis that affects approximately thirty-six million people. According to the Arthritis Foundation,one out of every seven Americans has arthritis, or inflammation of the joints. Victims have to change their activities and limit themselves because of pain. They need to learn about special types of exercises and where and how much to move. Arthritic inflammation is a disease that affects the whole body; it can produce swelling, stiffness, redness, and pain. Rheumatic diseases not only affect joints but also the muscles and connective tissues of the body. Only management through proper treatment can bring relief; there is no cure. Rheumatic diseases include fibrositis, low back strain, rheumatoid arthritis, ankylylitis, spondylitis, gout, osteoarthrosis, osteoarthritis, polymyadgia, rheumatica, and polymyositis.

The arthritis victim may become severely fatigued, especially if he suffers from rheumatoid arthritis and lupus. If this is the case, he must limit activities before he becomes tired. On the other hand, one may enjoy remission -- disappearance of symptoms -- or suffer flare-ups when pain is worse. The victim must learn to cope with this fluctuation and regulate his exercise accordingly. It is especially important not to push against pain, for this could cause further damage. One must be conscious that his needs are individual and the advice that his friend receives may not apply to him. It is possible for those with arthritis to overdo vigorous exercise and aggravate inflamed joints. If, after exercising, he feels pain in the joints that lasts two or more hours, he has done too much. He should make the distinction between therapeutic exercise and daily living movements, such as housework or yard work.

It is very important for the arthritic victim, through the advice of his physician or a physical therapist, to establish a prescribed program of exercise that includes both range of motion movements and strengthening movements.

Each joint can normally be moved a certain degree in various directions. This is known as range of motion exercise. Arthritis victims should take the time every day to try to move each joint through its complete range of motion to prevent stiffness and deformity. If this is done under the water, it is reasonably safe and comfortable.

Likewise, it is important to practice strengthening exercises, mostly isotonic resistive and isometric. If the joint is exercised against a weight or other resistance, such as water, it is isotonic resistive exercise. If a person strongly tightens a muscle but he does not move the joint, it is isometric, or muscle-setting exercise. The virtue of isometrics is that muscles can be strengthened without much actual joint motion.

Unlike most normal people, the arthritic victim should move slowly, steadily, and with rhythm that allows time for relaxing between repetitions of every exercise. Try to minimize stress on the joints, avoid high tension exercises (weight lifting) or extreme stretching. Try to alternate difficult activities with easier ones in order to minimize fatigue.

Allow for rest periods and make good use of flotation devices. Avoid tight grips on the side of the pool and distribute your weight evenly over several joints, for example, hold a ball or an object with the palms of the hands instead of the fingertips. Plan your exercise session so as to eliminate irritating exercises or those that are too demanding. Select exercises on the basis of strength development and range of motion. Always obey one rule: if it hurts, stop!

If at all possible use an indoor pool that has no drafts with 82° water temperature. Be sure to check with your doctor before you begin an exercise program, and supplement your exercise with proper diagnosis, education, medication, rest, good posture, proper diet and other aids. Contact the Arthritis Foundation, 1314 Spring Street, N.W., Atlanta, Georgia 30309, or your local chapter for periodical literature and Aquatic Programs. You must take the responsibility for your own well being by creating your own special lifestyle.

Charlie Byron, Chairman of the Physical Fitness for The Elderly Program of Connecticut's Department of Aging from 1970 to 1979, got his brown belt in karate in 1986, when he was 76 years old. Although he suffers from arthritis, he has adapted karate and katas movements so that they are beneficial because they are not jerky but flow rhythmically. He is dedicated to remaining active and helping others keep active and happy.*

Not only do Charlie Byron and other arthritic victims need to adjust their lifestyles and their exercises to their limitations, but so do countless diabetics, both Type I and Type II. According to The American Heritage Dictionary, diabetes is "a chronic disease of pancreatic origin, characterized by insulin deficiency, subsequent inability to utilize carbohydrates, excess sugar in the blood and urine, excessive thirst, hunger and urination, weakness, emaciation, imperfect combustion of fats resulting in acidosis, and without injection of insulin, eventual coma and death."

---

*Marjorie M. Dollar, "Charlie Byron: Coaching With A Heart," *Arthritis Today* (July-August, 1987), p. 6-8.

It is imperative for diabetics to consult with their physician or their diabetic advisor before they begin and while they participate in any exercise program. Except for serious heart diseases or problems, it likely is more of a matter of life and death that they take proper precautions than anyone else. During exercise the muscles use glucose for energy. Glucose in the blood and glycogen -- glucose that is stored in the liver and muscles -- are involved. After exercising, muscles continue to replace the stored glycogen that was burned, and replacing glycogen stores may take hours. This can seriously affect the body's glucose levels. In other words, when a diabetic exercises, the insulin in his last injection depot is drawn into the system while the glucose in the blood is being consumed by the exercising muscles. Thus a diabetic may experience dangerously low blood sugar during or after exercise if he does not carefully adjust his food and his dosage of insulin.

Yet exercise is valuable because the muscles use glucose with less insulin than they would otherwise. People with Type I (insulin dependent) diabetes may be able to reduce insulin intake if exercise is regular. Never reduce dosage without the physician's O.K.

Exercise can reduce blood-fat levels and help normalize blood pressure -- which lowers the risk of heart disease and arteriosclerosis. Aerobics are the best exercise for diabetics because they give the whole body a good workout. Most doctors advise thirty minutes of aerobics at least three times a week.

Side effects also must be considered, especially the site of the last injection of insulin. For example, if your last injection were in the thigh and you practice a lot of flutter kicking, the activity in the injected leg can make the insulin move into the blood at a faster than normal rate.

Special warnings and precautions are necessary. I am a Type I diabetic, and I never work out in the water without my "trusty jug." Not only am I guarding against low blood sugar, but also against dehydration. I fill my plastic bicycle jug with Tang. I like Tang because I can make it as weak or as strong as I desire. If I am going to lead an hour Aquacise Class and then swim one to two miles, I make the drink rather strong. If I am not going to be this active, I put very little Tang into the water.

Physicians and The American Diabetes Foundation* suggest more precautions. Never exercise when your blood sugar is over 240 and ketones are registered on your chemstrip. Always exercise after you have tested your blood accurately and after you have had a snack or a meal; your sugar is highest then. If your test result is less than 150, be sure to eat a snack before you exercise.

Check with your doctor to find out when your insulin peaks and do not exercise at that time. He may prescribe a special kind of insulin that will release slowly. Do not do isometric or heavy weight lifting exercises because they increase blood pressure and can damage your kidneys and your eyes. They can aggravate complications of high blood pressure. Always wear or carry a Medic-Alert identification. This can be critical in an emergency. If you ever have an insulin reaction, hypoglycemia

*American Diabetic Association, P. O. Box 2043, Mahopac, New York.

reaction, or an accident, people will know you are insulin dependent. The best ID bracelets give the phone number to identify your medication and whom to contact. Always keep glucose tablets, Life Savers, or a snack for emergencies. Let your lifeguard or someone at the pool know that you have diabetes. If possible, exercise or swim with a friend who knows how to recognize and treat hypoglycemia.

Do not overdo your exercise. If you have shortness of breath, intense sweating, a fast pulse or pounding heart that lasts for more than ten minutes after exertion, you have done too much. You also could feel exhaustion, insomnia or joint pains the day after a too heavy session. If you feel chest pain or pressure, severe shortness of breath, dizziness, nausea, stop immediately and call your doctor. You should avoid outdoor exercise in extreme weather. Do not smoke or drink caffeinated beverages for at least two hours before exercising. Drink fluids before, during and after a workout.

Whether or not you have diabetes or arthritis, you should be checked for hypertension and any cardiovascular disorder. You may have to avoid arm exercises because they raise your heart rate. Everyone should take a heart stress test and have a thorough physical examination before starting any kind of exercise program.

Do not think of growing older as growing weak or useless. Old is good. Ken Dychtwalk, known gerontologist, says that the older population in this country is rowing in power and impact.* They are vigorous, vital,

*"Growing Older and Better," *Arthritis Today,* I, No. 3 (May/June, 1987), p. 20-24.

attractive. For example, he praises Paul Newman and Joan Collins. In fact, it won't be very long until the Baby Boomers will be the Senior Boomers. Our average life span is expected to continue to grow. Only a hundred years ago the life expectancy was forty-five years and middle age was less than seventeen. Now the average life span is seventy-two. By the year 2000, the Rand Corporation predicts that the average life span will be ninety-two to ninety-six years.

Dychtwalk points out that the Baby Boomers (1946-1964), have interestingly matured from Dr. Spock's little rascals to creating a run on the education "industry," to becoming rebellious teens in the late sixties. They developed from Hippies to Yuppies, from flower children to conformists whose main center of interest is now work and making money. The seventy-six million Baby Boomers have matured and now they are beginning to age.

Not only the parents of the Baby Boomers, but the Boomers themselves, approach aging in a different way than ever before. Today senior citizens are active; they ignore the rocking chair. No longer is sixty-five the high water mark indicating old age. That was true in Europe a hundred years ago. Old age now begins at eighty or eighty-five. People no longer are thinking in terms of a single career followed by retirement. Some people who are in their seventies and eighties are starting new careers, maybe third or fourth careers. Our idea of glamour is associated with a forty-nine year old Jane Fonda, with forty-seven year old Raquel Welch and "ageless" Lena Horn."

People who have arthritis, who have diabetes, who have hypertension or heart conditions, even cancer, and all people who approach or are in their later years, are advised by medical authorities to be active, to have a regular program of exercise. The safest and best way to be active is to be an Aquaciser. The water prevents weight and stress on the feet and legs so that exercise does not aggravate varicose veins or foot problems as often do jogging or running. Deep breathing that is demanded in the water clears and develops the lungs and helps the whole cardiovascular system in a special way.

The "poor house" and the nursing home are being replaced by senior centers and by adult living areas where people may or may not garden or do domestic chores. Today we recognize the important differences between back breaking drudgery of housework and yard or farm work, and well directed exercise. No longer do informed people say, "I get enough exercise while I take a walk or do my housework." They may or may not do housework or necessary things, and then they go to a swimming pool for Aquacises -- for exercise, for its own sake, for the sake of their health, or just for fun! No longer do people pop pills; they pop into the water or onto a bicycle.

On the other hand, we all live in a world in which planes roars drown the news broadcast. We are bombarded by cars horns, by phones ringing, by the growl of vacuum sweepers and dishwashers, by endless and stupid chatter, and by "background music" in the doctor's and dentist's offices and in most television programs. If we become positively addicted we can get relief from stress of noise, of the Christmas season, of salesmen, of junk mail, of telephones, of automobiles and freeways, of organs and all that background music.

But what is *positive addiction** that can help us control our reactions to all the nonsense? It is the psychological condition or the state of mind that a person falls into as a result of doing something regularly several times a week that he does not have to do, but that he does for its own sake. It is a kind of peace, or maybe a shifting of the attention away from almost everything, and wool-gathering while you move or exercise. A common symptom of having PA is restlessness, even a sense of guilt or kind of withdrawal depression that happens if a person does not engage in the activity that created the PA state of mind.

Positive addiction, that results from exercise and not from yoga or meditation, has other characteristics also. The person who exercises reaches indirectly the state of mind that the meditators try to reach directly. For the athlete, PA is more a by-product than an end in itself. It increases one's self-confidence and improves the imagination. Basically, it is a private thing and it seldom is the product of a group activity. One rarely experiences PA in fewer than six months of regular exercise, regardless of the sport or the activity. It never is involved an competitive activities. You can not achieve PA by pushing for it or by trying to experience it. This effort could prevent your having PA at all. Simply let your mind spin free and you let PA happen.

---

*William Glasser, M.D., *Positive Addiction* (N.Y., Harper & Row Publishers, 1976), p. 145-46.

Just as negative addiction, such as alcoholism and drug addiction, over eating, etc., are passive by nature, positive addiction is the result of intense and repeated activity. Those who are most rewarded by achieving PA are those who have the self-discipline and strength to stick to a special activity. Such people make commitments to themselves that they will carry through their "thing" rather than find that they cannot accomplish anything unless they make a commitment to others. Unlike negative addiction, there is no reason to "kick" the activity because it has intrinsic value.

Dr. Glasser says that a person must, finally, experience the PA state regularly several times a week for several minutes to an hour each time in order to become addicted. Everyone can tap this magic.

Everyone, children, teenagers, Yuppies, seniors -- even post-seniors -- need to develop, maintain or restore their flexibility and vitality the fun way by enjoyable exercises with magical movement, rhythm, and dynamics.

Movement is fleeting like the notes of music. It seems to disappear instantly after it is created. It is the action that occurs between positions. Thus the illustrations and descriptions of exercises in this -- or in any other -- book can only hint at the movements you need to make, for only the isolated positions can be seen or captured for an isolated instant; it is impossible to capture "the given moment," even in music and ballet. Movement is a creative process that cannot be fully grasped because it is not fully tangible. Movement is a living process that involves the whole organism. Mere instructions, verbal or visual, cannot be a substitute for the physical experience, for the exhaustion, and the satisfaction. Movement is deeply personal and subjective. Make it your own.

Movement must be rhythmic and flow by creative energy through time and space. Think of your body as a musical instrument that plays silent magic. Make your movements rhythmic, the coordinated interplay of the dynamics of time and space. Rhythm is the order that regulates the sequences of movement, even of nature, life, and art.

All movement must have dynamics or force. The body must use increased energy while it keeps its balance, especially while it keeps its balance as it moves. Learn to feel your body use little energy when you allow gravity and momentum to help your movement. There is strong and soft, even heavy and light dynamics. Dynamics create stress, accent, increase or decrease tension -- it may be continuous or abrupt.

You can improve the movement, rhythm, dynamics of your body by conscious or kinesthetic awareness every time you do an exercise. Be form-conscious; also relax and let the water's resistance and your buoyancy help create the flow of movement.

The magical things, the best things in life, demand time: the aging of good wine; the writing and reading of great poetry; the composition and listening to great music; performing and seeing ballet; making love, and developing positive addiction through exercise. Creating and maintaining good physical and mental happiness and health are not the result of accidents or coincidence. They are, like other good things, the result of thought and of hard work. May everyone create magical living, and may Aquacises help others as it has and does help me. A better world has no alcoholics and many aqua-holics.

ETIQUETTE AND SAFETY

ETIQUETTE AND SAFETY

Regardless of where you go, whether it be a synagogue, a Catholic church, a mosque or a country club, certain behavior is expected. You do not have the same behavior and dress on the ski slopes or on a hike as you do at the opera. Conforming to expected behavior that is appropriate for the activity and the place makes things go smoothly for everybody.

Obedience to pool rules and appropriate etiquette is a matter of expediency and of safety. On the second page of the *American National Red Cross Lifesaving: Rescue and Water Safety,* are these words: "Disregard or ignorance of good safety practices ranks high in the cause of drownings. Regardless of swimming ability, a person must follow personal safety practices to be safe in the aquatic environment."

How many accidents - or near accidents -- on the highway have you seen that have been caused by bad manners? Using common courtesy is not simply civilized behavior, it is a method of survival. The first time you enter a swimming pool, ask about the rules and look around to see if they are posted. They should be.

If the rules are not posted, you can be sure that any good pool employee tries to enforce the following:

1. Walk. Do not run anywhere in the shower or pool areas. You could slip and get hurt.

2. Take a shower before you enter the water. A soap shower is preferred and it is required in many places. If you do not wear a hat, be sure that you shampoo your hair. Get perfume and spray net, etc. washed out.

3. Do not wear unhemmed cutoffs, shorts, or other non-swimming attire that could fray and clog filters.

4. Do not chew gum. You could choke to death on it. Do not smoke, and do not take food into the locker or pool areas.

5. Never wear street shoes in the pool or shower area. They carry all kinds of dirt and germs.

6. Always check to be sure that you dive into deep water; leave shallow starting dives to the experts.

7. Never jump or dive on other persons. Be sure the area is clear before you enter.

8. Do not interfere with lap swimmers. If you want to circle swim with someone in a crowded pool, ask the person(s) who are using that lane. Study the swimmers and match your pace to someone. Do not stop a swimmer who may be working on his time.

9. If you have a child with you, ask the guard if a swimming test is required before that child may enter deep water or use the diving board. Stay with your child and be responsible for his actions and his safety at all times. Lifeguards are not baby sitters. They watch everyone in the area.

10. Ask if children are permitted to wear masks or use toys or other equipment before you let the child use it.

11. If you have skin eruptions, sores, a cold or communicable disease, stay out.

12. Only one person at a time should be on either a diving board or ladder leading to a diving board.

13. Do not hang from the bottom of a springboard and do not take more than necessary bounce for a dive.

14. Do not distract the attention of, or enter into conversation with, a guard.

15. NEVER CALL FOR HELP UNLESS YOU NEED IT! In some places this results in a $500.00 fine or jail, or both.

16. Do not ask a guard to hold your valuables. Most places have lockers with keys. If there are no such provisions, put your valuables in your bag and place the bag out of the way on or near the deck where you can see it.

17. Never push, duck, shoulder stand, throw anyone, and do not take balls or toys into the pool.

18. Never bring glass bottles, glasses, soft drink cans, or any other sharp objects to pools or shower areas.

19. Stay out of the water when you are overly heated or immediately after eating.

20. Do not bring a child into the pool until his stool is hard, and use cloth, not paper, diapers.

21. Observe applicable, personal safety rules when you are swimming and at all other times.

If you will think about each of these rules, you can easily understand why you should observe them. If you are afraid of water, if you have any handicap, or if you want to understand something about the facility, be sure to speak with the cashier or an off-duty guard. Many non-swimmers can enjoy Aquacises and they may find added pleasure in devising their own exercises or new and different variations of those suggested in this text. The major objective is not that this book be read so much as it be used.

CONDITIONS THAT PROHIBIT EXERCISE

1. Any infectious disease during its acute state

2. Moderate to severe coronary heart disease that causes pain.

3. Recent heart attack. A three months waiting period is necessary before starting a regular conditioning program.

4. Obesity of more than thirty-five pounds overweight. First lose weight on a walking or moderate program and diet before beginning any strenuous jogging or exercise.

5. Severe disease of the heart valves, mainly the result of having rheumatic fever at an early age. Some victims should not exercise at all, not even walk rapidly.

6. Uncontrolled (by medication) high blood pressure; readings of 180/110 even with medication.

7. Special kinds of congenital heart disease in which the body's surface turns blue during exercise.

8. UNCONTROLLED sugar diabetes that may fluctuate between too much and to little blood sugar. People who do not test their blood before and after exercise on a daily basis.

9. Greatly enlarged heart that resulted from high blood pressure or other types of progressive heart disease.

10. Severe heartbeat irregularities requiring medication or frequent medical attention.

MEDICAL SUPERVISION NEEDED FOR EXERCISE

1. Diabetes (Type I) controlled by insulin.

2. Any infectious disease in its convalescent or chronic stage.

3. Convulsive disease not completely controlled by medication.

4. Internal bleeding recently or in the past. Get physician's O.K. to exercise.

5. Arthritis in the back, legs, feet or ankles that requires frequent medication to relieve pain.

6. Either chronic or acute kidney disease.

7. High blood pressure that can be reduced only to 150/90 with medication.

8. Uncorrected, but under treatment anemia.

9. Acute or chronic lung disease that causes breathing difficulty with light exercise.

10. Blood vessel disease of the legs that produces pain or ulcers.

EQUIPMENT

Like for almost every other sports activity, equipment may be simple and inexpensive or it may be complicated and costly. People usually are eager to sell something. You need only the basics, and even they are unnecessary (except for kickboards that are usually furnished by most pools) for Aquacising. A simple swim suit, a cap, and your own body are all you really need.

On the other hand, you may want to know about some other articles. Rubber bands, or approximately one inch wide rubber strips cut from an old inner tube are simple equipment. A strap is useful for imposing a handicap on yourself by twisting the band like a figure 8 and placing one ankle in each loop. Keeping your legs straight but relaxed, simply do the flutter kick, either by holding to the side of the pool, by using a kickboard, or by swimming. The band makes it difficult to spread your legs into a wide kick, and the effort you make in doing so is very beneficial. It feels great when you remove the bands!

A rubber covered, diving brick usually about ten pounds, also is helpful. Place the diving brick on one side and hold it with the top hand as you practice the side stroke. Ten pounds does not seem to be heavy, but as you practice, you will find that it seems to weigh tons. It also has other uses, among them is retrieving the brick from the bottom of deep water.

Pullbuoys are excellent devices for many things. Use them between the thighs to insure leg immobilization. A couple of times a week include a minimum of a non-stop half mile without kicking in a good workout. Using pull-buoys makes it easy to forget the legs that otherwise could not have enough buoyancy to drag well. This lets you concentrate on techniques of arm stroking. Pull-buoys are good teaching devices also. They offer slightly added water resistance in doing exercises.

Rubber balls are interesting for more than playing water games. You can place a ball near your rump, between the pool wall and your body. Then move your body in short vertical movements to roll the ball to your neck. You can hold the ball between your knees to do jumping and other exercises. Also, you can hold it between your hands as you do arm and bending movements.

Some of the most available and the most effective tools for adding resistance and handicaps to your exercising are old clothes. Old sneakers are especially useful for practicing kicks and leg exercises. When these old turkeys are wet, they are a real drag, and that is what you want.

Be sure that sneakers and old clothing are clean and free from soap and detergents when you use them in the pool. It is a mark of courtesy to ask the management's permission to use these things. Old T-shirts or sweat shirts, old jeans (hemmed), and socks are all good for practice work and exercising. The commercially made drag belt, that is worn just below the waistline, is popular for workouts among competitive swimmers.

Likewise, hand paddles are popular for swimmers' workouts. Paddles come in small, medium, large and extra large, and in several different styles and materials. They are excellent to use with pullbuoys for arm and shoulder workouts for the crawl -- and other stokes. Also, they are good for creating water resistance in performing arm exercises.

If you expect to remain in the water to swim or to exercise for long periods of time, goggles are really necessary. They protect your eyes against the sting of chemicals in pool water. They prevent your having that hazy or foggy eyesight after you have been swimming for a long time. Many doctors recommend that serious swimmers wear goggles.

Even though some doctors (non-athletic doctors) suggest wearing nose clips and ear plugs, *DO NOT USE EITHER OF THEM*. Nose clips are all right for some synchronized swimming, but for every other purpose they can be downright harmful. People who have never learned to breathe properly in the water use this kind of a crutch -- just as they often use masks and snorkels. Nose clips can cause problems with the eustachian tubes of the ear if one closes his mouth and swallows hard. After all, it is much simpler and a matter of common sense to simply get the habit of blowing some air or water out the nose instead of wearing the clips. Ear plugs are bad, mainly because they hold the water in the ear and prevent its naturally draining out, instead of being much good for keeping water out of ears. Only the baby-minded person can not get accustomed to some water in the ears. Expert aquatic people pull their caps so that their ears are exposed and the water can freely sift in and out of the ears. Some people put "Silly Putty" over children's ears or in their own if they have ear problems or infections. ***PEOPLE WITH INFECTIONS AND MEDICAL PROBLEMS SHOULD NOT BE IN THE POOL ANYWAY!***

Children and inexpert swimmers have no business using masks and/or snorkels. They prevent proper head rotation in water breathing and sometimes, if not manipulated properly, can cause suffocation. It is impossible to buy any equipment to substitute for skills.

One of the cheapest and best pieces of equipment for water exercises is an empty plastic vinegar or clorox bottle. Be sure that they are well rinsed before bringing them into the pool. Keeping most or all the air in the bottle, screw on the cap tightly. Hold a bottle by its handle in each hand and spread your arms and do some exercises. Many Aquacisers prefer the bottles to kickboards for most work.

Finally, unless you are a woman who carries a huge purse, it is a good idea to invest in a tote bag. A long bag is good; you can tuck fins inside it without any problems. All equipment is as long lasting and as good as the care it gets. Rinse your suit, cap, goggles, paddles, fins, etc. when you shower. Dry these things well with a towel and pack them evenly in your tote bag. Put your cap and suit into a plastic bag (grocery produce bag) so that the inside of your tote bag and other things stay relatively dry. As soon as you are home, hang your suit to dry and air your equipment. Before retiring at night, be sure that all equipment is nicely packed. Keep an extra swim suit and a towel, shampoo, conditioner, etc. in the bag ready to go at all times. If you keep your equipment in one bag, you will always have it with you and you will not have to search a dozen places to accumulate things.

Sharing a bag with a spouse can cause problems, mainly that of separate shower rooms for males and females makes it necessary for one of you to carry things in a towel. People who do not have organized containers for their equipment usually lose things. If you go on a trip, take your bag full of equipment, for there are fine places to swim throughout the United States, and especially in Canada. Now that you have a book full of Aquacises, suggestions, a sample plan, etc., you should have your fitness "in the bag."

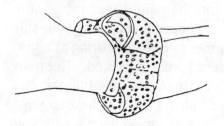

Swimmer's Drag Belt worn around the waist

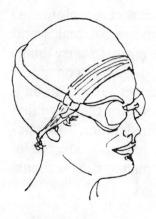

Swimmer's Goggles, prope worn over simple hat

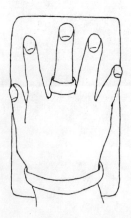

Swimmer's Hand Paddles

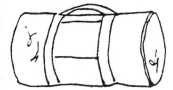

13" x 24" Handy Tote Bag

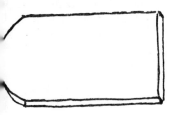

Regular sized KICKBOARDS are 12" x 24", and half sizes are 12" x 12". In addition to uses explained in this text is the board's value for support while practicing various kinds of kicks.

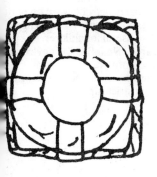

In addition to a RING BUOY and LINE'S being a key throwing assist for rescue, it is useful for towing poor kickers and gives beginners a feeling of water resistance. A proper buoy should be made of foam rubber, solid plastic, cork, or kapok. It weights about 2½ pounds. The rescue buoy usually has 50 feet of ¼ inch manila or polyethylene line attached to it.

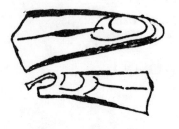

FINS are made in many sizes a
in various styles. I suggest usin
the full foot design, worn like a
shoe, rather than those that ar
open at the heel and are held
position by a heel strap. Some
fins float and others sink. It is
wise to wear socks under the f
until your feet are hardened b
using fins. Light, moderately
sized fins are best for exercise
purposes. Use of fins helps pe
fection of stroking, builds end
ance, and strengthens the legs
the back and stomach muscles

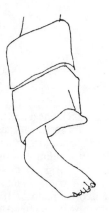

These are two FLOATERS*
worn on a leg as an anti-
gravitational device to enhanc
any or all of the water exercise
Floaters may be worn on both
arms and legs. Floaters likewi
are useful for children in a po
area. No inflatable device sho
be worn or used by non-
swimmers in open areas or wi
out strict supervision.

---

*Floaters are available at Belleair International, Inc.,
1016 Ponce de Leon Blvd., Belleair. FL 33516. Allegra Kent,
Water Beauty Book (N.Y.: St. Martin's Press, 1976), P. xii.

SUGGESTIONS FOR USING EQUIPMENT

BOTTLE EXERCISES

1. Keep the bottles under the arms. Stand up in water so that feet are free so as not to skin toes. Jog. Change to bicycling. Point your toes as your leg moves forward. Flex the ankle as the leg moves back.

2. In a sitting position with arms out, push legs forward and up to hip level. Keep the back straight. Flex the feet and make small circles. Point toes, split legs apart and then swing back at knees.

3. Lie in a back float with the bottles held out. Tighten all muscles. Keeping the body perfectly straight, swing the whole body down and forward into a front or standing float. Swing to back float and repeat.

4. You are standing in the water with your arms out. Lift the straight legs forward and up with the feet flexed. Tuck the knees to chest, then force down legs straight to toes and standing position again. Keep legs together throughout.

5. Lie on the back and float with legs together and arms out. Bend both knees to the chest. Kick legs forward. Make a splits wide apart. Pull legs straight together.

6. Lie in a vertical float and keep the bottles under the arms. Hold the feet together while bringing the heels toward the inside thigh. Lower feet to starting position. Hold feet together while bringing heels toward inner thigh. Split legs far apart and bring straight legs together. Bend the knees, soles of the feet together.

7. Sit with back straight, bottles under arms, heels under buttocks, feet flexed. Kick the left leg out to the side as you bring the right leg back to starting position. Kick the right leg out to the side. Alternate, kicking rapidly. Keep feet in the flexed position. Now, kick both legs forward at the same time. Repeat the series of movements several times.

8. Lie in a back float with bottles held out to the side. Bend the right knee up to the chest while the left leg is straight. Reverse so that you bend the left leg, and repeat alternately several times.

9. Lie in a back float with arms holding bottles out to sides. Roll onto the right side and scissors kick the legs apart. Do not pause. Roll onto the left side and scissors the legs apart and close legs. Roll right, scissors, close and repeat.

HAND PADDLE EXERCISES

1. Bend forward from the waist with the legs apart and straight. Turn the head to one side with arms out to the side. Tighten leg muscles and abdomen. Pull straight arms down and cross at the elbows in front of the knees. Push arms back up to the sides, body still moves from shoulders.

2. Your knees are bent, one forward and one back. Shoulders are wet and the arms extend forward at shoulder level forward at shoulder level. Backs of the hands touch, paddles turned out. Pull arms out and down in front of the abdomen and without stopping pull up to starting position. Reverse direction.

3. Knees are bent with one forward and one back. Arms are straight out to the side. Pelvic tilt. The straight arms trace large figure 8's out to the side. Paddles are in the direction of the swing. *Do not put stress on the back.*

4. Use the side split with arms out to the side and paddles forward. Twist at the waist. Turn to the left. Let the left knee bend, pivot on right foot until you are facing the opposite direction. *If you have lower back problems avoid this exercise.*

5. The knees are bent with one forward and one back; water should cover the shoulders; arms are straight, paddles face forward. Pull the arms together to center front. Push arms back out to the sides.

6. You are in a side split with water over the shoulders. Arms forward, paddles side by side. Both paddles

push against water to left side and then to the right side as the arms stay straight.

7. The knees are bent with one foward and one back as the shoulders are submerged and arms are out to the side with paddles forward. Pull the water forward, cross at the elbows in front of the chest. Push arms out to the side. Alternate upper arm as you repeat.

8. The knees are bent with one forward and one back. Shoulders are wet and arms are forward or at shoulder level with paddles turned down. Lean forward and push both arms behind you. Turn paddles down, lean back, and pull both arms forward and up.

PRINCIPLES FOR USING EXERCISE EQUIPMENT

BOTTLES

It is best to use bottles in deep water; however, never do so unless an instructor or a guard is closely watching if you can not swim.

Deep water is preferred for use of bottles so that your feet are free from the bottom and thus free from scraping.

If you are a non-swimmer and do not have an instructor, you might do similar or the same exercises on the wall.

Usually the bottle caps face forward as you hold bottles.

You can get various effects by putting different amounts of water into the bottles.

HAND PADDLES

People who have arthritis, bursitis, injury, etc. should probably avoid using hand paddles for exercises.

Use a pelvic tilt to keep the lower back from arching.

Keep the shoulders wet and use the paddles underwater.

TURN THE PALMS IN THE DIRECTION OF ARM MOVEMENT.

Keep a slight ease in the elbows and keep knees bent.

Change the forward leg every other time.

THIRTY MINUTE SAMPLE PLAN

WARM-UP

1. Trunk Twists - 15 times
2. Side Bends - 15 times
3. Elbow-to-Knee Touch
    a. Opposite - 10 times
    b. Same side - 10 times
4. Knee-to-Chest (alternate legs) 4 times
5. Body Bounce (forward, side, back, side)
6. Run with kickboard over head

JOGGING

In circles and across pool; change directions every 30 seconds.

WALL EXERCISES

1. Alternate Leg Touch - 10 times (back against wall)

2. Alternate Leg Jump - 2 sets of 30 seconds each

3. Sit-Ups (shoulders against wall, tuck and stretch) 20 times

4. Mule Kicks - 2 sets of 30 seconds each

5. Trunk Twists - 20 times (back to wall, one foot away, swing right and touch wall with both hands; swing left and touch wall with both hands)

6. Flutter Kick - sets of 30 seconds each

7. Bicycle Kick - 1¼ minutes (Shoulders against wall, go slow, medium, and fast)

8. Tuck and Stretch 5 times with each leg (Face wall, hands on gutter, knee to chin; then stretch behind)

9. Push-Ups (press aways) 15 times

10. Single Leg Lifts (forward, side, back - 5 times each direction with each leg)

AWAY FROM WALL - 2 kickboards

1. Shoot Through - 20 times; 10 open legs; 10 closed legs

2. Bicycle Kick - 1 min. (one board in each hand out to side, legs in front)

3. Rub-A-Dub-Dub - 15 times

AWAY FROM WALL - 1 kickboard

1. Board Boating - sit on board, 2 round trips across pool

2. Flutter Kick - 2 round trips across pool; hold board in front

3. Sit-Ups: 15 times (with board under arms and bend over board)

ON THE WALL WITH BOARD

1. Double Leg Lift - 5 times stomach; 5 times back (back and shoulders against wall, board between legs).

2. Trunk Twists - 20 times (shoulders against wall, board between legs, twist right to left to right)

AWAY FROM WALL

1. Arm Circles - 5 times forward and backward.   Shoulders wet.

2. Jumping Series

    a. Legs apart - 30 seconds (Jump up, bringing legs together, come down with legs apart)

    b. Legs together - 30 seconds (Jump up spreading legs apart; come down with legs together)

    c. Flutter Kick - 30 seconds (Jump up, flutter kick, come down, jump up, kick)

TAPER-OFF

1. Geometrical Arms
2. Arm pulls
3. Tip Toes
4. Rubber Neck
5. Waterpush

BIBLIOGRAPHY

Alexander, Ruth M. and Dorothy A. Shields. "Aquatics in Florida." *Journal of Health, Physical Education, Recreation.* XXXXIV. Jan. 1973. Pp. 83-84.

Allenbaugh, Naomi. "Learning About Movement." *NEA Journal.* LVI. March 1967. Pp. 48. 60. 64-65.

Anderson, Bob and Jean. *Stretching.* Published by the Andersons. Box 767, Palmer Lake, CA. Pp. 183.

Arthritis Aquatic Program: Guidelines and Procedures Manual. and *Arthritis Aquatic Program Instructor's Manual.* Atlanta, GA.: The Arthritis Foundation. 1983. Rev. Ed. Arthritis Foundation, Oregon Chapter. 1985.

Bailey, Covert. *Fat or Fit: A New Way to ealth and Fitness Through Nutrition and Aerobic Exercise.* Foreword by Joan Ullyot, M.D.. Boston, MA.: Houghton Mifflin Co. 1977. Pp. 107.

Barrett, Marcia et al, *Foundations for Movement. 2nd Ed.* Palo Alto, CA.: National Press Books. 1968.

Brown, Margaret C. and Betty K. Sommer. *Movement Education: Its Evolution and A Modern Approach.* Reading, MA.: Addison-Wesley. 1969. Pp. 260. Good gloss.

Casey, James Lynn. "Everybody Into The Pool." *Diabetes Forecast.* XXXX, No. 6. June, 1987. Pp. 50-52. Not recommended.

Cooper, Kenneth H. *Aerobics.* N.Y.: A Bantam Book pub. by arrangement with M. Evans & Co., Inc. 1968. Pp. x + 182.

Cooper, Kenneth H. & Mildred. *Aerobics for Women.* N.Y.: A Bantam Book, pub. by arrangement with M. Evans & Co., Inc. 1973. Pp. 160.

Cooper, Kenneth H. *The Aerobics Way.* N.Y.: A Bantam Book, pub. by arrangement with M. Evans & Co., Inc. 1977. Pp. 31I.

Cooper, Kenneth H. *The New Aerobics.* N.Y.: A Bantam Book, pub. by arrangement with M. Evans & Co., Inc. 1970. Pp. 171 + appendix & bibl.

Councilman, James E. *The Science of Swimming.* Englewood Cliffs, N.J.: Prentice-Hall,Inc. 1968. Pp. xiii + 457.

Dake, Debbie. *Dancercize.* Englewood Cliffs, N.J.: Prentice-Hall, Inc. 1967. Pp. 190.

Dollar, Marjorie M. "Charlie Byron: Coaching With A Heart." *Arthritis Today.* July-Aug. 1987. Pp. 6-8.

Duffield, M. H. *Exercise in Water.* London: Bailliere Tindall. 1967.

Duke, Deirdre J. and Robert A. Gianguzsi.. "Exercise for The Elderly." *Diabetes Self-Management.* Jan/Feb. 1987. Pp. 10-14. Excellent article.

Gardiner, M. Dena. *The Principles of Exercise Therapy.* London: G. Bell & Sons Ltd. 1953. Pp. xi + 260.

Ginsberg-Fellner, Fredda. "Balancing the Scales: Weight Control for Teens Is A Delicate Problem." *Countdown: Juvenile Diabetes Foundation International.* VIII. No. 3. Sept., 1987. Pp. 22.

Glasser, William. *Positive Addiction.* N.Y.: Harper & Row Publishers. 1976. Pp. 4+159.

"Growing Older... and Better." *Arthritis Today,* I. No. 3. May-June, 1987. Pp. 20-24.

Holmer, Ingvar. "Psychiology of Swimming Man." *Exercise and Sports Sciences* Review. VII. 1979.

"How Exercise Helps." *Diabetes '87: The Newsletter for People Who Live With Diabetes.* Summer Issue. The American Diabetes Association, P.O. Box 2043, Mahopac, N.Y. 10541.

Ishmael, William, and Howard B. Shorbe. *Care of the Neck.* Philadelphia, PA.: J. B. Lippincott Co. 1966. Pp. 20. Not recommended.

Kelly, Ellen Davis. *Adapted and Corrective Physical Education. 4th Ed.* N.Y.: The Ronald Press Co. 1965. Pp. vii + 350.

Kent, Allegra. *Water Beauty Book.* Introd. by Edward Villella. Photos by Martha Swope. N.Y.: St. Martin's Press. 1976. Pp. xii + 163.

King, Frances & William F. Herzig. *Golden Age Exercises.* N.Y.: Crown Publishers. 1968. Pp. ix + 134.

Krewer, Semyon. *The Arthritis Exercise Book.* N.Y.: Simon & Schuster. 1981.

Lifeguard Training. Washington, D.C.: The American National Red Cross. 1983.

Lifesaving, Rescue, and Water Safety. Prepared by The American National Red Cross. Garden City, N.Y.: Doubleday & Co., Inc. 1977. Pp. 10 + 240.

Kubssley, Ruth, Billie J. Jones, and Ada Van Whitely. *Body Mechanics.* Dubuque, IA,: William A, Brown, Co. 1970.

Lustgarten, Karen, Photography by Bernie Lustgarten. *The Complete Guide To A Dynamic Body.* N.Y.: Fawcett Columbine Books, A Unit of CBS Publications. 1980. Pp. 160.

Lurie, Jesse Zel and Samuel Segev, Eds. *The Israel Army Physical Fitness Book.* N.Y.; Grosset & Dunlap. 1969. Pp. 128.

Midgley, Ruth and Hope Cohen, Eds. *The Complete Encyclopedia of Exercises: Select and Vary Your Individual Routine With This Illustrated Step-by-Step Guide to More Than 350 Different Exercises.* N.Y.: Grosset & Dunlap. 1979. Pp. 335.

Mitchell, Curtis. "Tone Up The Swimming-Pool Way." *Family Health Magazine.* July, 1970.

Morehouse, Lawrence and John Cooper. *Kinesiology.* St. Louis, Mo.: C.V. Mosby Co. 1950.

Perlow, Nat, Ed. *Water Exercises.* Greenwich & Stamford, CT.: Globe Communications Corp. 1979. Pp. 64.

"Rules To Live By." *Diabetes '87: The Newsletter for People Who Live With Diabetes.* Spring Issue. The American Diabetes Association. P.O. Box 2043, Mahopac, N.Y. 10541.

Sholtis, M.G. *Swimnastics is Fun.* Washington, D.C.:American Alliance for Health Physical Education and Recreation, a HPER Publication. 1975. Pp. vii + 38.

Sterling, Barbara. *Aquatics for The Handicapped.* N.Y.: Hoffman-Harris. 1958.

Swimming and Aquatics Safety. Washington, D.C. The American National Red Cross. 1981. Also all other Red Cross publications.

Especially Important:

Adapted Aquatics with 165 Illustrations. N.Y.: Doubleday & Co., Inc. 1977. Pp. 11 + 254. This is the finest source for aquatics and the handicapped.

All Issues of the Following Periodicals

American Journal of Occupational Therapy

Arthritis Today

Countdown: Juvenile Diabetes Foundation International

Diabetes Forecast

Diabetes Newsletter

Diabetes Self-Management

Journal of The Association for Physical and Mental Rehabilitation

Journal of Health, Physical Educaton and Recreation

Swimming Technique

Swimming World and The Junior Swimmer

Recreation

Cover design by Lyrl Ahern.

Illustrations by author.

Photo of author by Mary Burns, A. F. Ph.

Printed and bound by Little River Press, Inc.,

Miami, FL.

Other Books from Mills & Sanderson

Winning Tactics for Women Over Forty: How to Take Charge of Your Life and Have Fun Doing It by Anne DeSola Cardoza and Mavis B. Sutton. A multi-faceted guide for those women now in their forties and fifties who have suddenly found themselves having to adapt their lifestyles to a world for which they were not prepared. Explicit chapters cover such essentials as health, personal growth, adapting to loss, financial planning, housing options, etc. The connections, techniques, resources and options available to these women are extensively covered. **$9.95**

Aquacises: Restoring and Maintaining Mobility with Water Exercises by Miriam Study Giles. Unlike most of the exercise books presently available. Aquacises is devoted to both the physical and psychological fitness of those millions who just want to feel better—and move around better in their normal activities. Written by a former dancer who has taught swimming and exercise for more than half a century, this book is primarily focused on senior citizens' needs, but is also an invaluable resource for those suffering from physical handicaps and those too self-conscious about their shapes to join in community calisthenics. **$9.95**

There ARE Babies to Adopt: A Resource Guide for Prospective Parents by Christine A. Adamec. Author-researcher Adamec, an adoptive parent herself, provides a tremendous amount of valuable information and advice aimed at helping you adopt the baby you want. Gleaned from both personal experience and in-depth interviews with over a hundred other adoptive parents, social workers, and other adoption specialists, this practical guidebook dispels the popular myth that there are no healthy babies available for adoption unless you are willing to wait five to seven years. **$9.95**

Fifty and Fired! How to Prepare for It; What to Do When It Happens by Ed Brandt with Leonard Corwen. The authors lead the middle-aged, middle-manager through the trauma of age motivated job dismissal using actual hard-hitting case histories to show what can be done before and after the fact to defend your career and dignity, and rebuild your livelihood. **$9.95**

Your Astrological Guide to Fitness by Eva Shaw. Find out what your astrological sign has to say about your ideal exercises, sports, and menus. There are also astrologically keyed gift ideas and comparison charts to help you choose your ideal mate or traveling companion. **$9.95**

Bachelor in The Kitchen: Beyond Bologna and Cheese by Gordon Haskett with Wendy Haskett. From Beer Jello to Duck with Cherries, San Diego chef Gordon Haskett shows you quick and easy recipes for yourself and/or that special someone in your life; also, how to be the hit of any party or Pot Luck. **$7.95**

60-Second Shiatzu: How to Energize, Erase Pain, and Conquer Tension in One Minute by Eva Shaw. The author explains how acupressure relief can be self-administered amidst the frustrations of commuter rush hours, college exams, family fights, or office hassles. It's fun, it's easy, and it works! **$7.95**

Smart Travel: Trade Secrets for Getting There in Style at Little Cost or Effort by Martin Blinder. The author's thirty years of globe-spanning travel have taught him many secrets for getting the best of everything for as little expense as feasible, and he wants to share those secrets with you. **$9.95**

The Cruise Answer Book: A Comprehensive Guide to the Ships and Ports of North America by Charlanne F. Herring. This book offers a tremendous amount of information about ships, itineraries, shore excursions, and ports that is not included in other cruise guides, and that will help you decide which cruise is best for you at any particular time. This book concentrates on cruises around North America, the Caribbean, Bermuda, Hawaii...the areas where most Americans choose to cruise. **$9.95**

Adventure Traveling: Where the Packaged Tours Won't Take You by T.J. "Tex" Hill. Whether you're looking for the keen edge of real danger or trips that invoke the tingle without the threat, here's an international menu of itineraries and guidelines for the vacationer who is looking for a "different" kind of vacation. **$9.95**

Order Form

If you are unable to find our books in your local bookstore, you may order them directly from us. Please enclose check or money order for amount of purchase plus handling charge of $1.00 per book.

( ) Winning Tactics for Women Over Forty @$9.95 _____

( ) Aquacises @$9.95 _____

( ) There ARE Babies to Adopt @$9.95 _____

( ) Fifty and Fired! @$9.95 _____

( ) Your Astrological Guide to Fitness @$9.95 _____

( ) Bachelor in The Kitchen @$7.95 _____

( ) 60-Second Shiatzu @$7.95 _____

( ) Smart Travel @$9.95 _____

( ) The Cruise Answer Book @$9.95 _____

( ) Adventure Traveling @$9.95 _____

    Add $1.00 per book handling charge _____

    Add 5% Sales Tax if MA resident _____

    Total Amount enclosed _____

Name _____

Address _____

City/State/Zip_____

Mail to: Mills & Sanderson, Publishers
       442 Marrett Road, Suite 5
       Lexington, MA 02173